the 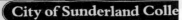 ok

CD Books

Habia – RELATED TITLES

HAIRDRESSING

Start Hairdressing! – The Official Guide to Level 1 *Martin Green and Leo Palladino*
Hairdressing: The Foundations – The Official Guide to Level 2 *Leo Palladino*
Men's Hairdressing: Traditional and Modern Barbering *Maurice Lister*
African-Caribbean Hairdressing *Sandra Gittens*
Salon Management *Martin Green*
Mahogany: Steps to Cutting, Colouring and Finishing Hair *Martin Gannon and Richard Thompson*
Mahogany Hairdressing: Advanced Looks *Martin Gannon and Richard Thompson*
Patrick Cameron: Dressing Long Hair *Patrick Cameron and Jackie Wadeson*
Patrick Cameron: Dressing Long Hair Book 2 *Patrick Cameron*
Bridal Hair *Pat Dixon and Jacki Wadeson*
Trevor Sorbie: Visions in Hair *Trevor Sorbie, Kris Sorbie and Jackie Wadeson*
The Total Look: The Style Guide for Hair and Make-Up Professionals *Ian Mistlin*
The Art of Hair Colouring *David Adams and Jacki Wadeson*

BEAUTY THERAPY

Beauty Therapy: The Foundations – The Official Guide to Level 2 *Lorraine Nordmann*
Professional Beauty Therapy – The Official Guide to Level 3 *Lorraine Nordmann, Lorraine Appleyard and Pamela Linforth*
Aromatherapy for the Beauty Therapist *Valerie Worwood*
Indian Head Massage *Muriel Burnham-Airey and Adele O'Keefe*
The Complete Nail Technician *Marian Newman*
Safety in the Salon *Elaine Almond*

the colour book

THE OFFICIAL GUIDE TO COLOUR
FOR NVQ LEVELS 2 AND 3

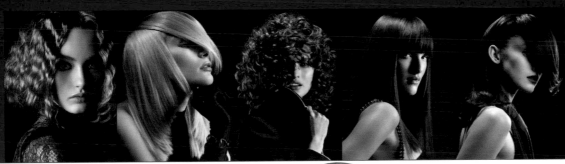

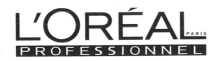

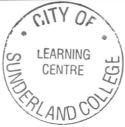

TRACEY LLOYD
WITH CHRISTINE MCMILLAN-BODELL

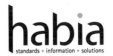
standards · information · solutions

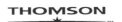

Australia · Canada · Mexico · Singapore · Spain · United Kingdom · United States

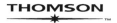

The Colour Book: The Official Guide to Colour for NVQ Levels 2&3
Tracey Lloyd with Christine McMillan-Bodell

Publishing Director John Yates	**Manufacturing Manager** Helen Mason	**Marketing Manager** Natasha Giraudel
Production Editor Alissa Chappell	**Production Controller** Maeve Healy	**Illustrations in Chapters 1, 2 and 6** Oxford Designers and Illustrators
Typesetter Meridian Colour Repro Ltd	**Text Design** Design Delux, Bath, UK	
Cover Design Ruth Stanley, Silverstone	**Development Editor** Melody Woollard	**Printer** G Canale & C, Italy
Publisher Lib Wright		

ISBN-13: 978-1844-80141-1
ISBN-10: 1-844-80141-1

This edition published 2005 by Thomson Learning.

British Library Cataloguing-in-Publication Data
A catalogue record for this book is available from the British Library

contents

dedication

I would like to dedicate this book to my best friend Michelle who is always there and knows this book almost as well as I do! Also, to my beautiful son Alfie who lights up my world with his smile and is the best motivator in the world.

Tracey Lloyd

what can The Colour Book do for you?

Chances are, if you are a level 2 hairdressing student, you have already realised how exciting it will be to be able to colour hair to a professional standard. You will soon be equipped with the skills and know-how to make a great cut look even better, how to enhance a client's best features and bring out their individual style.

If you are at level 3, you will no doubt be looking forward to taking your colour knowledge even further to master more advanced techniques and achieve even better colour results. You will be able to provide expert colour services to those clients that need their hairdresser to help them to achieve their dream look.

Whether at level 2 or 3, The Colour Book and its accompanying interactive CD-ROM will help you to learn the colour skills you need to send your clients away looking and feeling fantastic but it has also been written with your formal qualification in mind. You will find that everything you need to complete your colour related NVQ units at levels 2 and 3 have been covered in detail with plenty of glossy step by step photos, expert tips, fun activities and much more. You will find more useful information about colour and your NVQ and how you can make the most of this complete course companion in About the book, page xi.

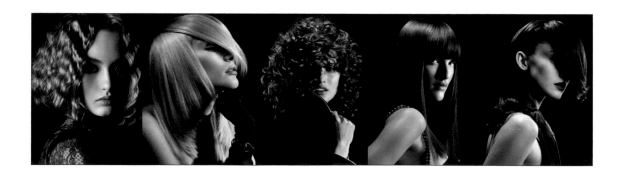

acknowledgements

I would like to thank Lib Wright and Melody Woollard for all their support and guidance during the writing and production of this book. It has been a unique experience and would not have been completed without your constant encouragement and patience. Thank you.

Tracey Lloyd

The publisher and L'Oréal Professionnel would very much like to thank Christine Hillyer-Smith, Education Development Co-Ordinator for L'Oréal Professionnel, for her expertise in the field of hair colour. Her work specialises on the animation of colour education to tutors of NVQ, helping them to deliver the best quality colour education, whilst providing the industry with the next generation of highly qualified colour specialists able to reach their full potential.

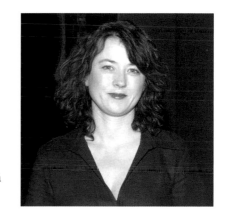

Thanks also to Rena Valez at Central Saint Martins College of Art and Design for her contribution to the chapter introductions.

Thomson Learning and *L'Oréal Professionnel*

Habia foreword

The past few years have been extraordinary for hairdressing, in terms of growth, fashions, styles and trends.

Nowhere has that been more evident than in hair colouring.

Such is the growing demand for colouring, even amongst men, that it is one of the most vital and sought after salon skills.

As a result there is a need for a book that encompasses the entire world of hair colouring in all its shades and textures, and helps those just starting out or looking to upgrade their skills to meet this much in-demand service.

This vibrant and informative book displays the world of hair colour in its full glory, covering all its aspects in a comprehensive yet easy to follow way.

But what really makes this book work so well is the knowledge and experience of the authors.

Tracey Lloyd has nearly 25 years' experience of hairdressing, in the UK and internationally, and has dedicated herself to passing on her knowledge through education. With a background as a course leader and an internal verifier, Tracey's commitment to learning shines through in this informative book.

Likewise, Christine McMillan-Bodell also has nearly 25 years' hairdressing experience, with 20 of those years in education. Having worked as a lecturer, course leader and internal verifier, Christine is ideally placed to develop and design methods of learning that are effective and inspiring, as can be seen in *The Colour Book*.

Both Tracey and Christine are authorities in their field, and have created a book that even the most seasoned and experienced professionals will find of interest.

I have every confidence *The Colour Book* will prove an invaluable resource to students, salon professionals and salon owners alike.

Alan Goldsbro
Habia CEO

about the book

This book relates to the NVQ/SVQ Levels 2 and 3 qualification structure and to the current Habia (Hairdressing and Beauty Industry Authority) national occupational standards for hairdressing. It offers full coverage of the following colour related units:

- H13 Change hair colour using basic techniques (Level 2)
- H28 Provide colour correction services (Level 3)
- H30 Colour hair using a variety of techniques (Level 3)

However, all great hair colourists will need to be effective when consulting with their clients, remain aware of health and safety in the salon and know how to contribute to the smooth running of the salon in general, so the book covers the following units too:

- G1 Ensure your own actions reduce risks to health and safety (Levels 2 and 3)
- G6 Promote additional products and services to clients (Levels 2 and 3)
- G7 Advise and consult with clients (Level 2)
- G9 Provide hairdressing consultation services (Level 3)
- G11 Contribute to the financial effectiveness of the business (Level 3)

Finally:

- Chapter 1, *The Colours of Life*, provides coverage and all required knowledge of anatomy and physiology for hairdressing at levels 2 and 3
- Chapter 7, *Technique Matters*, is packed full of step by step guides from L'Oréal Professionnel – the world number one for hair colour, to help you create a variety of exciting looks and styles using your colour knowledge.

FEATURES WITHIN CHAPTERS

Each chapter is packed full of lively examples and full colour illustrations plus the following carefully constructed features to aid your learning process:

Learning objectives

Learning objectives introduce each chapter and provide a run down of what that chapter will cover and the units it relates to.

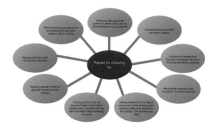

Spidergrams

Spidergrams are provided to summarise the skills and knowledge requirement for the elements of the various units covered throughout the book. You'll find that they provide a handy checklist when revising.

ACTIVITY

Furthering the conversation
Think of three ways that you can move the client conversation forward.

Activity boxes

Activity boxes provide additional tasks for you to complete to further your understanding of the unit. Some of them, if completed correctly, may even count towards your portfolio.

TIP ✓

Following manufacturer's instructions, temporary colour products can be used to brighten existing tones.

Tip boxes

The author's experience is shared in the tip boxes. You will find plenty of positive suggestions to help you improve your knowledge and skills for each unit and when working in the salon.

HEALTH AND SAFETY +

Always make sure you protect yourself when applying a semi-permanent colour by wearing suitable disposable gloves and an apron.

Health and safety boxes

Chapter 6, *You and Health and Safety in The Salon* covers health and safety in the salon in detail but health and safety boxes are also found within the other chapters to help to draw your attention to related information and considerations for the technical units.

Case study

For example:
Your client has Majirel 5.52
on her hair =   Depth of 5 Light brown
                       Primary tone .5 = Mahogany (cool)
                       Secondary tone .2 = Ash iridescent (cool)
Is this a warm or cool mahogany?
Your client has Majirel 4.56
on her hair =   Depth of 4 Brown
                       Primary tone .5 = Mahogany (cool)
                       Secondary tone .6 = Red (warm)
Is this a warm or cool mahogany?

Case studies

Case studies provide a practical opportunity for you to practice your colour knowledge.

Assessment of knowledge and understanding

Each chapter ends with a thorough assessment of knowledge and understanding for you to complete. Each question relates to the specific essential knowledge and understanding requirements for each unit. You can use these questions to prepare for your oral and written assignments.

CD-ROM symbols

Where any part of the book is further explored on the accompanying interactive learning CD-ROM, you will find a symbol in the margin telling you if an activity, or video clips are available on the CD-ROM. See About the CD-ROM for further information.

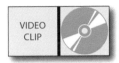

Assessment of knowledge and understanding

Test yourself on the content of this chapter by answering these questions. This will help you to prepare for your Essential knowledge/Written test.

1. What are the different types of protective equipment available? Explain why it is important to use personal protective equipment.

2. Why is it important to position your colouring tools and equipment so that they are easier for you to use?

3. What are the safety considerations that you must carry out when you are colouring hair?

4. Give two reasons why work areas should be kept and left clean and tidy.

5. Why is it essential to have good personal hygiene?

6. Why should you always check electrical equipment before you use it?

7. Give two reasons for the importance of following manufacturer's instructions when using colouring products.

8. Draw and describe three line diagrams demonstrating how temporary, semi-permanent and quasi-permanent (tone on tone) colours affect the hair structure, including how long each colour product lasts.

VIDEO CLIP

A porosity test

Step by step photos

Each colour application procedure for the colour units listed are illustrated in clear, full colour step by step photos with easy to follow instructions along with step by step photos and instructions on how to complete the related hair and skin allergy tests. Many step by step sequences are further explored in video clips on the CD-ROM – look out for the CD-ROM symbols.

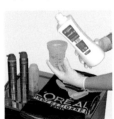

1. Equipment required for application

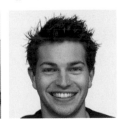

2. Mix product as directed

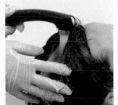

7. Spread evenly through hair

8. Continue with application

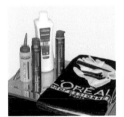

3. Measure required oxidant

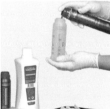

4. Before colour application

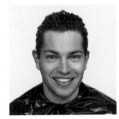

9. Leave for full development time

10. Add water to emulsify and rinse

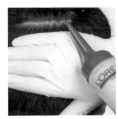

5. Section the hair to start application

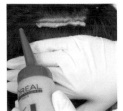

6. Begin application at root area

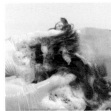

11. Shampoo gently

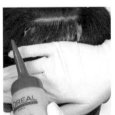
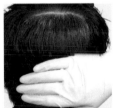

12. Final result

about the CD-ROM

A unique interactive learning CD-ROM accompanies The Colour Book. It allows you to step into a virtual salon and expand your colour skills. Key features of the CD-ROM include:

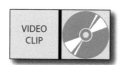

Video clips

Video clips are provided to bring to life some of the colour applications shown in the step by step photos in the book.

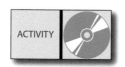

Animations and Activities

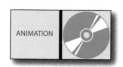

Animated diagrams and activities provide a practical demonstration of various topics such as the science of the hair and skin, colour correction and hair and skin allergy testing.

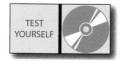

Self testing

Question and answer screens give you the opportunity to self-test as you gain your colour knowledge, and help you to prepare for assessments.

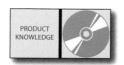

Virtual product library

A selection of colour products are stored in the virtual product library allowing you to enhance your product knowledge and to practice selecting everything you would need to carry out colour applications.

'My Portfolio'

'My Portfolio' lets you save your work for your tutor or supervisor, for future reference, or even to count towards your final assessment.

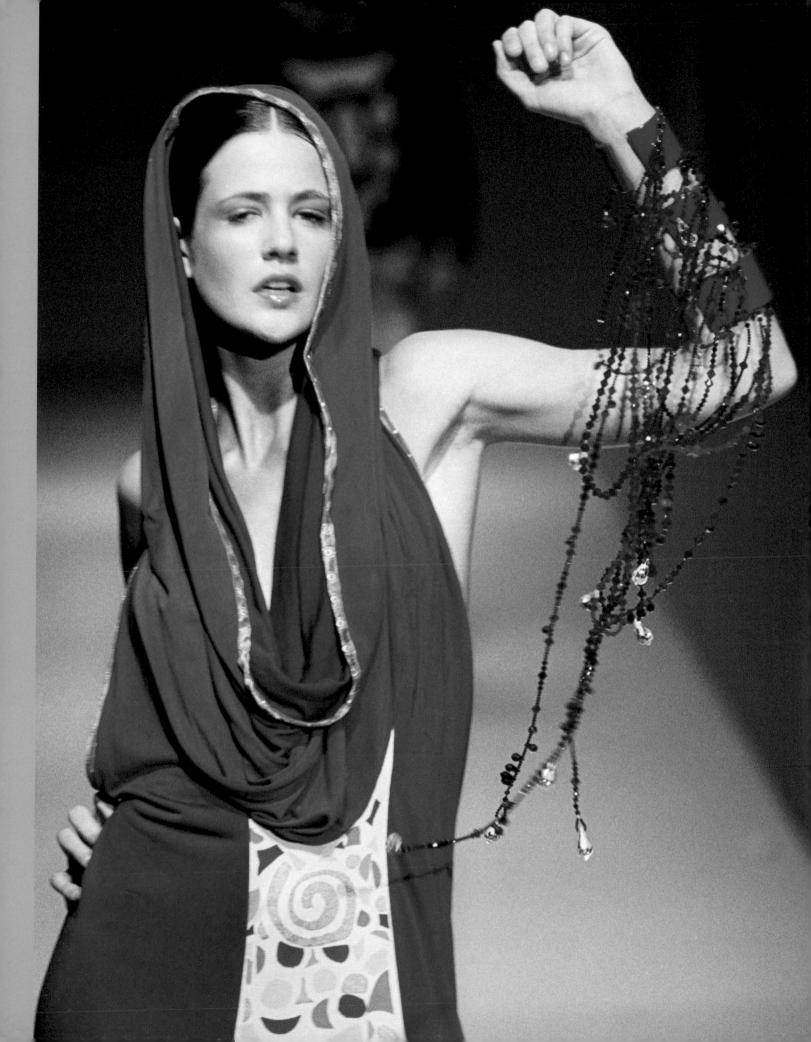

The colours of life

In ancient Rome, the formula for black hair dye consisted of leeches and vinegar left to ferment in a lead container for two months. If you wanted to colour your hair red for a wild night out, you'd reach for the goat fat and beechwood ashes. Blondes had more fun, or at least more fragrance, with a recipe of ashes, nutshells and elderberries that sounds like the vegetarian option in quite a few restaurants today.

The ancient Egyptians used henna – a red plant-based dye – and indigo. To the dark-haired Romans, the fair hair of the conquered Teutons (ancestors of modern day Germans) was exotic, so blonde hair was a sign of beauty. They bleached their hair with saffron, red arsenic, nutshells and plant ashes.

Historically, the appeal of blondes is based on little more than physical health. When disease was common among much of the population and medical practice was based largely on magic and superstition, skin tone was an outward sign of good or ill health. The fair skin of blondes was more difficult to disguise, so it was easier to tell if a potential spouse was healthy or not.

Fortunately, things have changed since then! Leeches are difficult to find in your local pharmacy and department stores are clean out of lead containers, especially around Christmastime. Not to mention that most of us don't want to smell like a chip shop anyway.

The lengths to which people would go to achieve the hair colour they wanted tells us how important colour is in our lives – how it looks, the effect it has on our mood, what it says about us. It's part of our language, both verbal and visual. We see red, go green with envy, feel blue when things aren't going well.

Colour is thought to have therapeutic properties, and colour therapy and healing are now part of complementary medicine. In the eighteenth century, Quaker hospitals were painted green because the colour appeared to have a calming effect on patients.

Our fascination with colour is found in every civilisation and culture, throughout the ages. Early cave painters mixed natural materials to create colours. These, often incredibly sophisticated, paintings date to around 12000 BC: even then, humans were experimenting with colour to leave their mark on the world.

We've always wanted to be able to change or improve the way we look and make-up and hair colour are part of our history, signifying status, tribe, class, political allegiance, wealth and of course, fashion and beauty.

Now, here we are in the twenty-first century and almost anything goes. You can look how you want, when you want. However, until the nineteenth century, men's hair and clothes were as elaborate as women's. Portraits from the seventeenth century show men in luxuriant wigs and in the eighteenth century, men powdered their wigs with a rainbow of colours.

Throughout the nineteenth century, many tints were unpredictable and often dangerous to the skin, and hair colouring was usually a hit and miss affair. In 1907, a French researcher named Eugene Schueller recognised the need for safe and effective hair colours and created the first scientifically-based hair tints. He registered the name Aureale which later became L'Oréal, now a globally recognised brand.

Beauty preparations advanced after the Second World War when fashion, including hair style and colour, became less rigid. With the introduction of temporary colour sprays and hair colours for home use, nearly one woman in five was using hair colour by the beginning of the 1950s.

In the 1960s, the status of hairdressers was transformed and they became celebrities. Once the backroom girls and boys, they are now the story and often the stars. A salon's prestige once came through its clients: now clients acquire prestige and profile by going to the 'right' hairdresser.

Colour makes life exciting. It calms us, stimulates us, make us more – and sometimes less – attractive, and makes our world a richer place. Through advances in colour technology, we now have access to colours that previously did not exist.

Colourists will always be in demand. It's a career that can take you around the world. Great colourists will always be an integral part of the film, music and fashion industries. If the idea of a less hectic life appeals, the local salon, and perhaps eventually your own business, is a great way to make a living. Whichever way you look at it, there's never been a more exciting time to be a colourist.

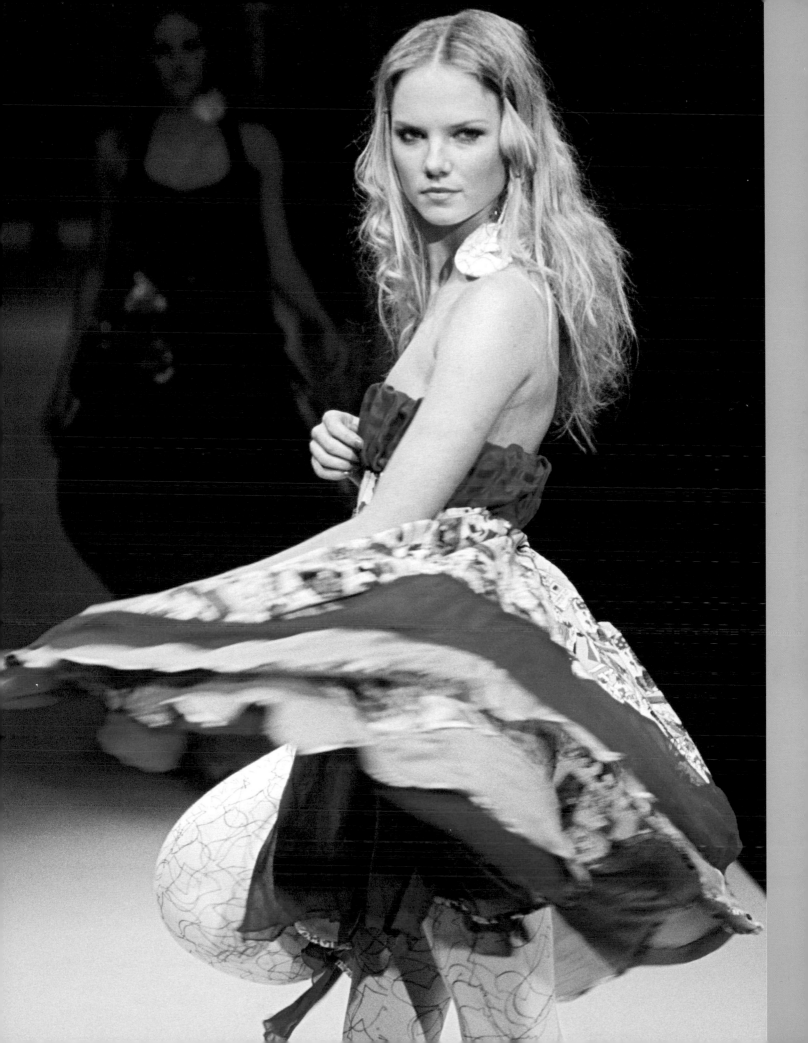

chapter 1

THE COLOURS OF LIFE

Learning objectives

This chapter will provide you with the foundations to build on for your future colour knowledge. In *the colours of life*, we will consider:

- **The structure of the hair and skin**
- **Porosity, sensitivity and elasticity of the hair**
- **The hair growth cycle**
- **The primary colours**
- **How hair gets its natural colour**
- **Natural depths of colour**
- **Natural lightening**
- **Artificial lightening**

THE STRUCTURE OF THE HAIR AND SKIN

Our hair protects the scalp and head from the elements and helps us to retain body heat. Before we look at colour theory, you need to understand the way hair and skin works.

The structure of the skin

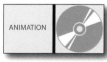

The structure of the skin

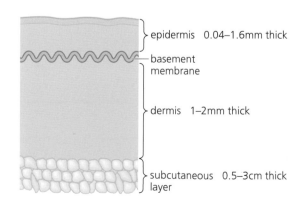

epidermis 0.04–1.6mm thick

basement membrane

dermis 1–2mm thick

subcutaneous layer 0.5–3cm thick

The structure of the skin

The structure of the skin

The skin structure consists of three distinct layers:

- The epidermis layer
- The dermis layer
- The subcutaneous layer.

Epidermis

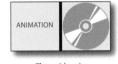

ANIMATION

The epidermis

The epidermis is the skin's shield: the skin that you can see and touch. It helps to protect us from outside attacks such as bacteria, viruses and temperature changes. The epidermis is very thin and is made up of many layers. Depending on its location around the body, it can vary in depth from 0.04mm up to 1.6mm. For example, the soles of the feet have a thick layer, while the eyelids are very thin and delicate.

The epidermis and its many layers

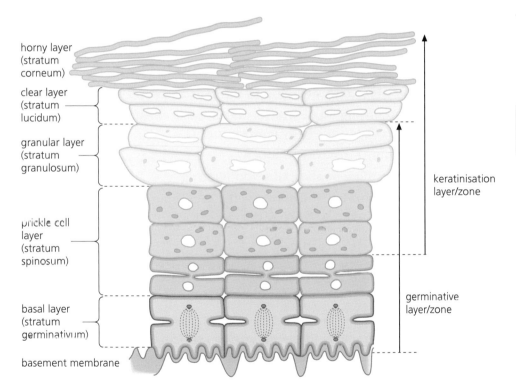

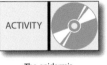

ACTIVITY

The epidermis

Dermis

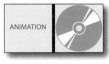

ANIMATION

The dermis

The dermis, or true skin, which consists of a fibrous tissue is 1 to 2 mm thick, forms the framework of the skin. Contained within the dermis are the blood vessels, nerves, the arrector pili muscles and the sebaceous and sweat glands.

The dermis

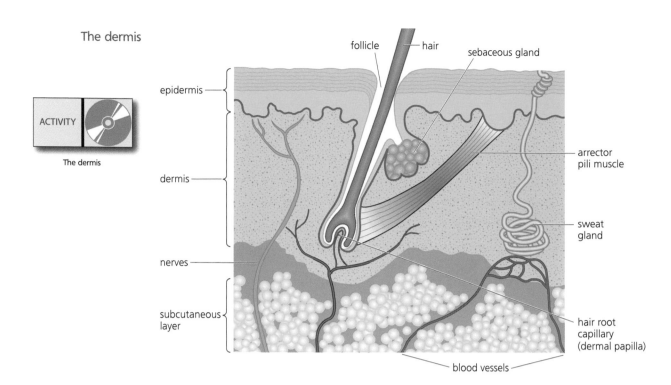

The components of the dermis are responsible for:

- Blood vessels – Providing nutrition to the cells and epidermis
- Sweat glands – Storing water which is released as sweat when we are hot: this helps to regulate your body temperature
- Nerves – Providing sensitivity to touch
- Epidermis – Providing permeability and filtering
- Blood vessels – Providing nutrition for the sebaceous glands and the dermal papilla.

Subcutaneous layer

Beneath the dermis is the fatty subcutaneous layer which firmly attaches the skin to the scalp, merging with the dermis, the subcutaneous tissue acts as insulation to prevent the loss of body heat.

The hair follicle

The hair follicle itself is an extension of the germinative layer; at its base is the dermal papilla where the hair is formed in an area called the matrix. Each cell divides, creating another cell which is pushed upwards by the birth of other cells. They keratinise (harden) progressively in the top part of the hair root thus producing the hair.

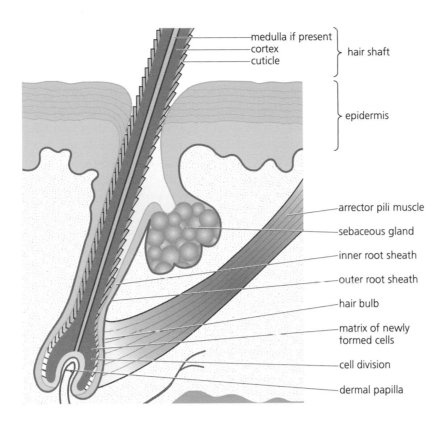

A cross-section of the hair follicle and hair

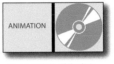

Cross-section of the hair follicle

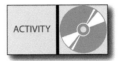

Cross-section of the hair follicle

The structure of the hair

Hair is produced from a protein called keratin in the dermal papilla. As the cells are pushed upwards they undergo changes; degenerating, elongating (getting longer), they lose their nucleus (their centre) as they gradually harden and die. Therefore hair that you can see and touch is dead, but it will retain elasticity due to its chemical structure. As the cells elongate they intertwine and start to form the three layers of the hair shaft, the cuticle, cortex and medulla.

It is also during this process that the hair's natural pigment is deposited by melanocytes producing melanin. We will look at these pigments later in the chapter.

The structure of the hair consists of three layers:

- The cuticle
- The cortex
- The medulla.

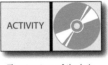

The structure of the hair

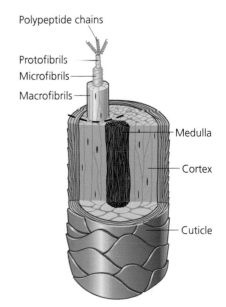

The structure of the hair

The cuticle

The cuticle is the protective surface of the hair and is located on the outside of the hair shaft (see the illustration, 'The structure of the hair' on page 9). It consists of a single layer of cells which partly overlap, in a similar way to fish scales or tiles on a roof. As the scales overlap each other several times, a cross-section of the cuticle gives the impression of there being a multilayered structure, with 3–10 layers of thickness. The cuticle is translucent which means that light passes through the scales, giving it a reflective quality. (Think of a frosted window where the light shining through is diffused but no definite shape can be seen.) The cuticle plays a very important role, contributing to the consistency of the hair and keeping the keratin fibres of the cortex within a sheath that is very stable and resistant to physical and chemical forces. When the cuticle deteriorates, it loses its protective powers and the internal cohesion of the hair is reduced, so the hair becomes considerably more fragile.

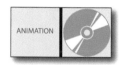

The cuticle showing porosity and elasticity tests

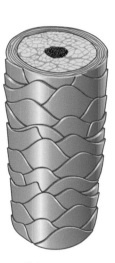

A healthy cuticle

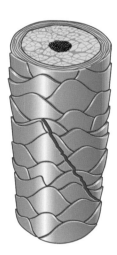

A damaged cuticle

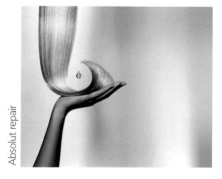

Healthy hair should be smooth and shiny

Conditions affecting the cuticle

Porous hair

When the hair is in good condition the cuticle lays flat to the hair shaft, reflecting light and creating shine and vitality: it will feel smooth and compact to touch. When the hair is in bad condition, the cuticle scales are raised and the hair does not reflect the light as effectively, giving it a dull, lifeless appearance: it will feel rough to the touch. When the cuticle is in this state, we call this porous hair. Hair will accept chemicals more readily if it is in a porous condition.

Suitable steps must be taken to ensure that artificial colour remains in the hair and does not escape through the open porous scales.

The porosity of the hair is affected by the following during and after the colouration procedure:

- Sun and wind
- Electrical equipment such as hair straighteners and hairdryers
- Chemical products
- Salt water or chlorinated water.

How to test for porosity

Step 1 Take a few strands of hair and hold firmly near the points

Step 2 Slide your fingers down towards the roots

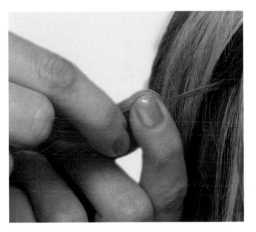

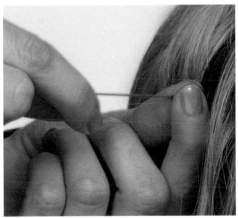

Step 1

Step 2

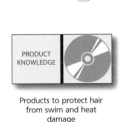

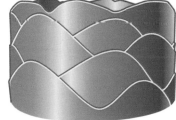

Products to protect hair from swim and heat damage

Step 3 The rougher and more swollen the hair feels, the more porous its condition.

Pre-colour and post-colour treatments will help to even out the porosity level of the hair. Deep-acting treatments will penetrate into the cortex giving suppleness and moisture to the fibres as well as smoothing the surface cuticle.

The cortex

The cortex of the hair has an absorbent sponge-like consistency and contains the hair's natural colour or pigments. (See How does hair get its natural colour?, p. 18) Any chemical changes take place within the cortex, including those caused by artificial colouring and lightening or perming and relaxers. Keratin cells that are located in the centre of the hair follicle take the shape of tapered spindles or keratin chains; these constitute the heart of the cortex. When the bonds of the keratin chains are intact the hair will be strong, if the bonds break the hair will become weaker.

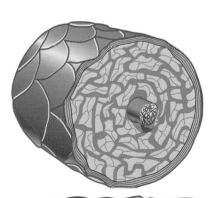

The cortex

The keratin chains or tapered spindles are composed of small bundles of:

- Cortical cells
- Macrofibrils
- Microfibrils
- Protofibrils.

Cortical cells

The cortex contains cortical cells; these are sealed to each other and run in the same direction as the hair shaft. They are approximately 100 micrometres in length and are made from a series of cells called macrofibrils.

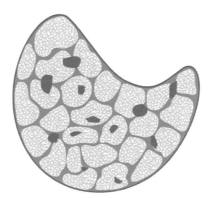

One cortical cell

Macrofibrils

The macrofibrils contain granular pigments of melanin which are responsible for your natural hair colour. These cells consist of microfibrils which are covered with a formless matter rich in sulphur and in turn form even smaller bundles of microfibrils.

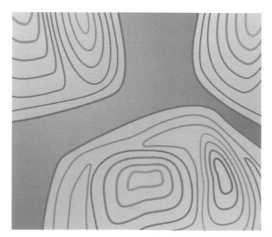

Macrofibrils

Microfibrils

The structure of the microfibrils consists of the combination of 5–11 protofibrils.

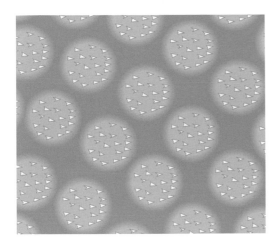

Microfibrils

Protofibrils and keratin chains (polypeptide chains)

The protofibrils make the keratin chains. When two or three of these chains are grouped together they take on the form of a protofibril and are held together in alignment at the centre of the cortex by chemical, disulphide, hydrogenous and saline bonds. These bonds provide cohesion for this complex structure. The presence of a protein component called intercellular cement will ensure that the keratin chains are protected at all times.

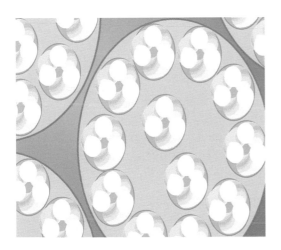

Protofibrils

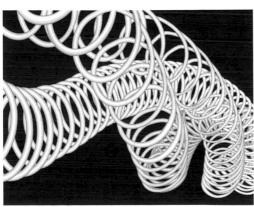

Keratin chains

Introducing conditions affecting the cortex

Hair sensitivity and its causes

When the hair becomes damaged at the level of the keratin chains it is likely that it will not return to its original length and shape once stretched.

This is caused by:

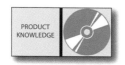

Product to protect hair from heat damage

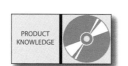

Product to protect hair from swim damage

- Electrical damage – using heated equipment such as hairdryers and hair straighteners on a regular basis
- Excessive chemical services – for example double processing without following manufacturer's insructions
- Naturally weak hair (lack of cystine, an essential amino acid) – this could be due to poor health or if the client is taking medication
- Salt/chlorinated water, excessive sun – for example a client who swims regularly in a public swimming bath or someone who has just come back from a holiday in the sun.

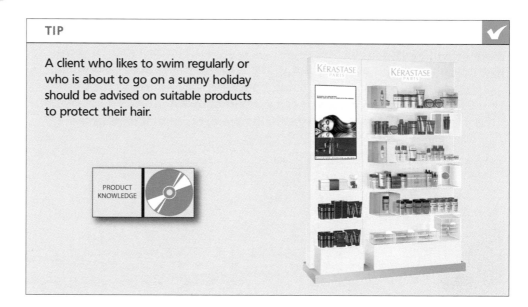

TIP

A client who likes to swim regularly or who is about to go on a sunny holiday should be advised on suitable products to protect their hair.

When the hair has been subject to damage the intercellular cement will break down causing the keratin chains of the hair to be weakened. (The intercellular cement of the hair is a natural protein which acts as a glue-like secretion, helping to hold all of the cells in the hair in place, including the alignment of the keratin chains.) If this happens, essential amino acids will be lost and the bonds which link the chains together will be weakened or broken causing the hair to lose its strength.

Sensitivity, like porosity, is nearly always uneven according to the age of the hair and the amount of abuse it has encountered. It is important for us to be able to recognise the signs of sensitivity and porosity when colouring the hair as it can have a dramatic effect on the results we achieve. During client consultation the strength of each individual hair is tested by the use of an elasticity test (you are testing the strength within the cortex) and the overall diameter or texture of the hair shaft plays an important part in choosing the most appropriate treatment for the client's hair.

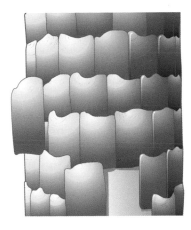

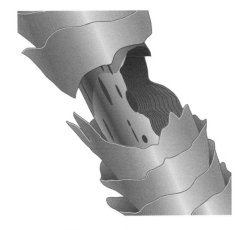

Normal hair is shiny and smooth with the intercellular cement intact

Hair with intercellular cement cracked and missing

How to test for elasticity

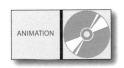

ANIMATION

Elasticity test

The strength and elasticity of the hair are extremely important to us as hairdressers. When the hair is in good condition and the bonds are strong the hair will be able to stretch one-third of its original length and return: hair in poor condition is often unable to do this.

Step 1 Take a single damp hair, holding it between two fingers, with wrists together, gently stretch the hair

Step 2 It should stretch and return to its original length

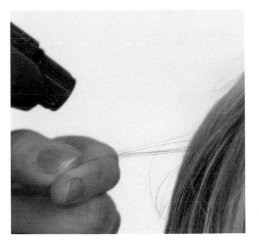

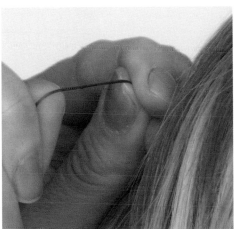

Step 1

Step 2

Step 3 When elasticity is lost the hair will not return to its original shape.

Naturally sensitised hair

This can sometimes occur due to a lack of the essential amino acid, cystine, in the hair, although the hair may appear to be in good condition.

The medulla

The medulla is like a straw running centrally through the hair and has been found to serve no purpose in the hair structure itself. There can be many air spaces along its length and in some cases the medulla is missing or only present at intermittent places along the length, this is dependent on the texture of the client's hair. The medulla plays no part in any chemical process or non-chemical treatments in hairdressing. In many animals it is no longer present in the hair, and theories suggest that through evolution it will also eventually disappear in humans.

The medulla
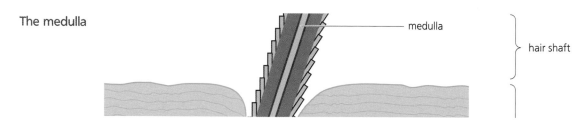

THE HAIR GROWTH CYCLE

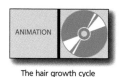

The hair growth cycle

Hair has a continuous life cycle of growing and falling out: each individual hair reaches a different stage at a different time so there is continuous renewal and replacement of old hair for between two and seven years.

The hair growth cycle

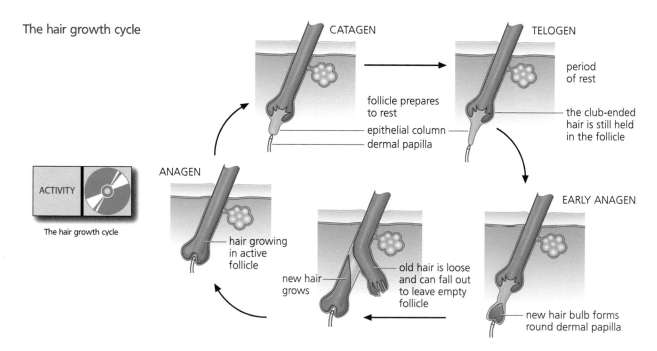

The hair growth cycle

Anagen

This is the active stage of the growth cycle and signifies growth within the papilla and germinal matrix. It is at this stage that the hair's texture, shape and colour is formed. Hair in this stage can grow from a couple of months up to several years. Hair growth rate is about 1.25 cm or half an inch per month.

Catagen

At the end of the growth period of the anagen cycle, the hair stops growing and the hair bulb becomes gradually separated from the papilla. The hair bulb begins to break down and the follicle begins to get shorter. This phase lasts for about two weeks.

Telogen

The follicle now enters a resting stage where no growth occurs. This stage lasts from a few hours up to around four months. After this time, the follicle lengthens again and a new bulb forms around the original papilla. Towards the end of the telogen stage, cells begin to activate in preparation for the new anagen stage of growth.

The new hair starts to grow and the old hair is pushed out. This old hair is often seen in combs and brushes and you can expect between 100–150 hairs per day to naturally fall out of the scalp.

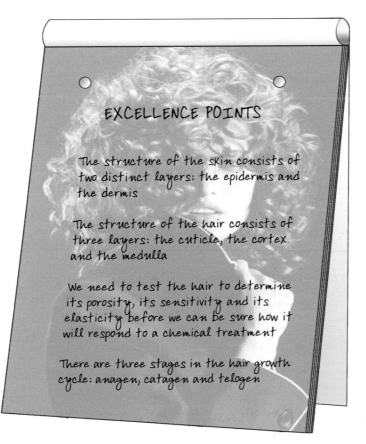

EXCELLENCE POINTS

The structure of the skin consists of two distinct layers: the epidermis and the dermis

The structure of the hair consists of three layers: the cuticle, the cortex and the medulla

We need to test the hair to determine its porosity, its sensitivity and its elasticity before we can be sure how it will respond to a chemical treatment

There are three stages in the hair growth cycle: anagen, catagen and telogen

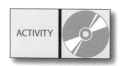

ACTIVITY

The primary colours

PRIMARY COLOURS

Any colour in nature, however it is reproduced, is a mixture of blue, red and yellow. These three colours are called 'primary colours' or 'colours of life'.

Mixing primary colours

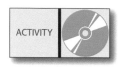

ACTIVITY

The secondary colours

When you superimpose (place on top of one another) or mix together these three primary colours, they give all the known shades, from the darkest to the most pastel. There are millions of shades you can make but when mixed together in equal quantities they always give us brown. When you mix primary colours together as shown below they will produce *secondary* or *complementary* colours, therefore:

Blue + red	purple
Red + yellow	orange
Yellow + blue	green

HOW DOES HAIR GET ITS NATURAL COLOUR?

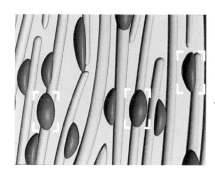

Granular pigment

Hair gets its natural colour from the two pigments that are contained within the cortex of the hair:

- Granular, more commonly know as melanin, pigments
- Diffused, more commonly known as pheomelanin pigments.

Granular (melanin) pigments are quite big and dark: from blackish to light brown, everyone has them. They are composed of all the primary colours: blue, red and yellow.

Diffused (pheomelanin) pigments are tiny, and spread out everywhere in the cortex of the hair, they are essentially yellow and infused throughout: everyone has them.

Therefore, whether the hair is brown or light blonde, it contains the same pigments but in varying quantities. So if we all have these pigments in our hair, why do we all have different coloured hair? Because different quantities and combinations of these pigments give us different hair colours: it is the *quantity* of each pigment that will determine your hair colour.

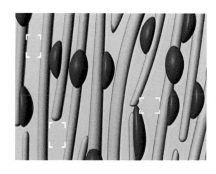

Diffused pigment

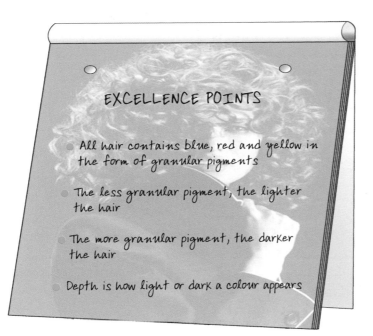

EXCELLENCE POINTS

- All hair contains blue, red and yellow in the form of granular pigments

- The less granular pigment, the lighter the hair

- The more granular pigment, the darker the hair

- Depth is how light or dark a colour appears

NATURAL DEPTH

Depth is how light or dark a colour appears. As we have learnt, all hair contains blue, red and yellow in the form of granular and diffused pigments. Each individual has hair which makes him or her totally unique. Remember that the less granular pigment the lighter the hair, the more granular pigment the darker the hair.

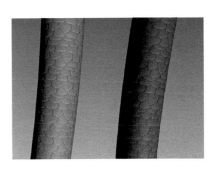

Natural hair

TIP ✔
Most natural depths fall between 1–9. It is very unusual to find a natural depth of 10 on a client.

Range of depths

The depths range from 10 – Lightest blonde to 1 – Black. The International Colour Code (ICC) sets out natural depths into the following categories:

10 – Lightest blonde

9 – Very light blonde

8 – Light blonde

7 – Blonde

6 – Dark blonde

5 – Light brown

4 – Brown

3 – Dark brown

2 – Darkest brown

1 – Black

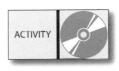

ACTIVITY

Levels of colour

We will look at the International Colour Code in more detail in Chapter 3, Commit to colour.

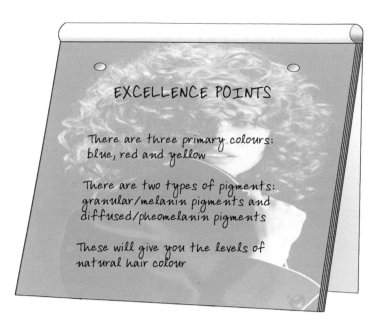

EXCELLENCE POINTS

There are three primary colours:
blue, red and yellow

There are two types of pigments:
granular/melanin pigments and
diffused/pheomelanin pigments

These will give you the levels of
natural hair colour

NATURAL LIGHTENING

Natural lightening of hair occurs when the hair is exposed to oxygen in the air. This natural lightening process will be accelerated when you expose your hair to sunlight. Humidity that is carried in the atmosphere by the wind also carries the oxygen to the hair, which will help to increase the natural lightening process. Oxygen first attacks the granular pigments; the blue is the weakest and virtually disappears. As they oxidise, the pigments change colour to expose the naturally warm tones of the hair. For example, dark hair will expose red tones after being in the sun.

Therefore, oxygen will naturally lighten your hair!

| Humidity | = Wind/air = oxygen | Oxygen lightens the hair. |
| Sun | = UV rays | Heat from the sun accelerates this process. |

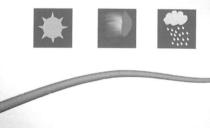

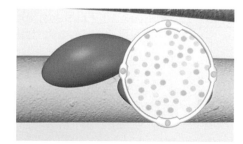

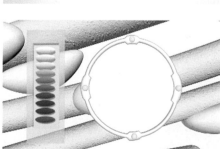

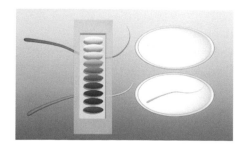

ARTIFICIAL LIGHTENING

When we artificially lighten hair with chemical products concentrated oxygen is present, giving a much more powerful effect within a controlled development time.

When bleaching (pre-lightening) products are applied, granular (melanin) pigments lose their blue particles, then red and orange, before they finally turn yellow. These 'transition' colours are called 'levels of lightening' or 'undercoats'.

In a second phase, the oxygen affects the diffused pigment (pheomelanin) which is yellow and more resistant to the oxidation process.

The transition from yellow to pale yellow often requires stronger ingredients and oxidants. You can see this change of colour during highlighting when using bleaching (pre-lightening) products.

If you try to lighten the hair too much you will destroy its inner strength, so be cautious when trying to achieve a very light base and always follow the manufacturer's instructions.

The undercoats

When you artificially lighten the natural hair pigments you create an undercoat.

The L'Oréal Professionnel levels of lightening chart below can be used as a guide when lightening to estimate the undercoat colour at each depth. For example: 7 blonde = yellow orange.

Levels of lightening chart

Depth No.	Depth Name	Pigment	Level of lightening
10	Lightest Blonde		Very Pale Yellow
9	Very light Blonde		Pale Yellow
8	Light Blonde		Yellow
7	Blonde		Yellow Orange
6	Dark Blonde		Orange
5	Light Brown		Orange Red
4	Brown		Red
3	Dark Brown		Red
2	Darkest Brown		Red
1	Black		Red

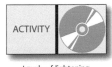

Levels of lightening

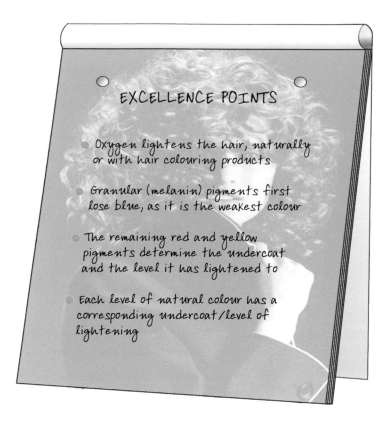

EXCELLENCE POINTS

- Oxygen lightens the hair, naturally or with hair colouring products

- Granular (melanin) pigments first lose blue, as it is the weakest colour

- The remaining red and yellow pigments determine the undercoat and the level it has lightened to

- Each level of natural colour has a corresponding undercoat/level of lightening

Case study

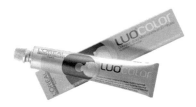

Now that you know the depths and undercoats, use the case studies below to see what would happen if you went two shades lighter than your natural depth? What would your new depth and undercoat be?

1 Natural depth 6 – Dark blonde taken two levels lighter would result in being, 8 – Light blonde with an undercoat of yellow

2 Natural depth 4 – Brown taken two levels lighter would result in being, 6 – Dark blonde with an undercoat of orange

ACTIVITY

Now you know the principle of using the levels of lightening chart, using your colleagues as clients assess their existing depth and undercoat and imagine they would like to be two shades lighter. What would their new depth and undercoat be?

You now know the principles of how to artificially lighten hair and this knowledge is a good basic start for you to be able to work with pre-lightening products. Please refer to Chapter 3 for application techniques, product knowledge, working safely with bleaching (pre-lightening) products and further information on this subject. Good luck!

Assessment of knowledge and understanding

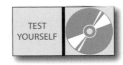

TEST
YOURSELF

Testing and essential
knowledge

Test yourself on the content of this chapter by answering these questions. This will help you to prepare for your Essential knowledge/Written test.

1 How many layers is the skin structure made of and what are they called?

2 What is the base of the hair follicle called?

3 What protein is hair made from?

4 Draw and label the different parts of the hair structure.

5 What different elements cause porosity?

6 How do you test for porosity?

7 Name the different chains contained within the cortex.

8 Approximately how far can the hair stretch when it is in good condition?

9 How can you damage the cortex of the hair?

10 How do you test for elasticity?

11 Describe each stage of the hair growth cycle.

12 What are the three primary colours?

13 Name the colours that are produced when you mix primary colours together.

14 What is the natural colour pigment called?

15 Describe granular (melanin) and diffused pigments (pheomelanin) in terms of size and quantity.

16 Describe the term colour depth.

17 Name the range of colour depths as stated in the ICC numbering system.

18 What can naturally lighten your hair?

19 Describe how you would artificially lighten your hair.

20 What is described as an undercoat?

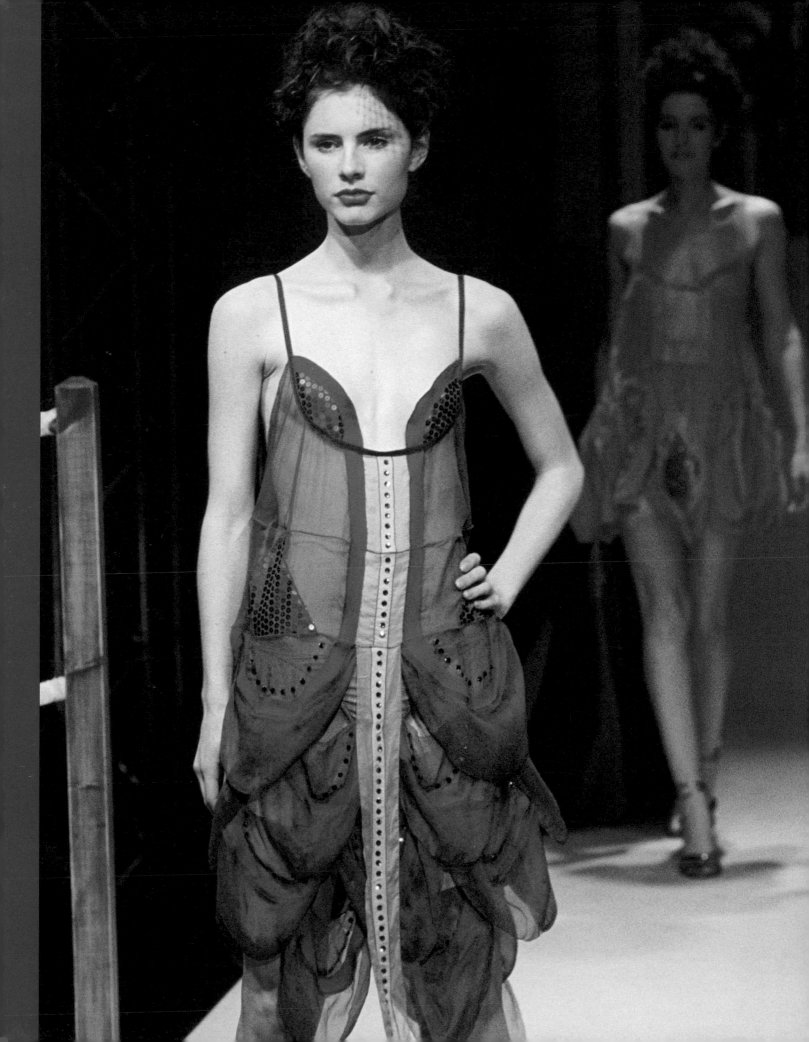

No-commitment colour

Tweed is in. Green is the new black. Boots are just so last week. Fashions change – and while we may not change our hair colour as often as we change our shoes, fashion influences our cut and colour to create a total look.

Magazines tell us what we're going to be wearing next season, but how do they make their predictions? The spring/summer and autumn/winter ready-to-wear catwalk collections in Paris, London, Milan and New York are the major influences on the choices we make.

The key trends in cut, shape, and colour in clothes, make-up and hair that come out of the shows will dominate magazines and press for the next six months.

Often, the collections of different designers will have a similar look or theme. So have they all had the same idea, but interpreted individually? People talk of the 'spirit of the times' and fashion designers get their inspiration from film, music, popular culture, television and the street. In fact, like anyone creative, inspiration can come from anywhere at any time. The difference is in what they do with it. And it's the sense of what's coming next that keeps us all fascinated.

chapter 2

NO-COMMITMENT COLOUR

Learning objectives

This chapter will teach you how to add colour to hair using temporary, semi-permanent, quasi-permanent and organic products. In this chapter. In *no-commitment colour* we will consider:

- **Adding colour to hair using temporary hair colour products**
- **Adding colour to hair using semi-permanent hair colour products**
- **Adding colour to hair using quasi-permanent (tone on tone) hair colour products**
- **Adding colour to hair using organic hair colour products**
- **How different factors such as porosity, percentage of white hair, and different types of hair can affect the colour result**
- **How to protect yourself and your client when providing temporay, semi-permanent, quasi-permanent and organic colour treatments**

H13 Change natural hair colour using basic techniques

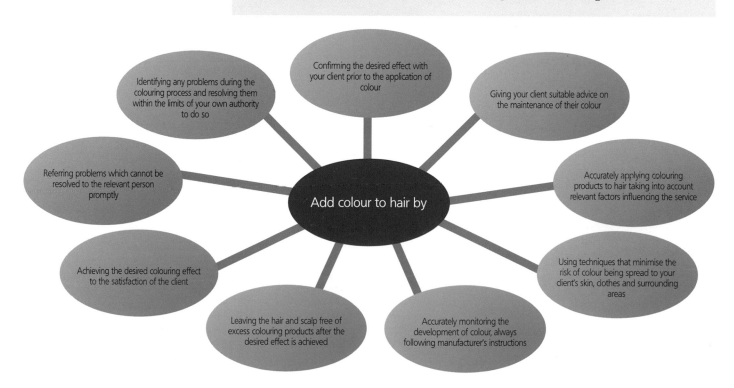

Identifying any problems during the colouring process and resolving them within the limits of your own authority to do so

Confirming the desired effect with your client prior to the application of colour

Giving your client suitable advice on the maintenance of their colour

Referring problems which cannot be resolved to the relevant person promptly

Add colour to hair by

Accurately applying colouring products to hair taking into account relevant factors influencing the service

Achieving the desired colouring effect to the satisfaction of the client

Using techniques that minimise the risk of colour being spread to your client's skin, clothes and surrounding areas

Leaving the hair and scalp free of excess colouring products after the desired effect is achieved

Accurately monitoring the development of colour, always following manufacturer's instructions

TEMPORARY COLOUR

Although they are still used, for some time temporary colours have been regarded as an old fashioned and outdated concept in the hairdressing industry but you need only go into your local hairdressing suppliers to see a whole new generation of vibrant and fashionable temporary products. Temporary colours need no development time and come in many different forms such as setting lotions, mousses, colour sprays and colour shampoos.

TIP ✓

Following manufacturers' instructions, temporary colour products can be used to brighten existing tones.

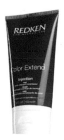 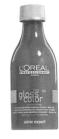 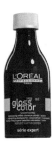 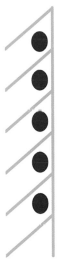 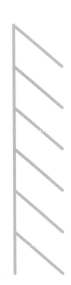

Why would we use a temporary colour on a client's hair?

- To introduce your client to hair colouring
- To produce short-term fashion effects
- To temporarily restore hair to its natural colour
- To neutralise unwanted yellow tones in bleached (pre-lightened) or yellow hair

What different types are there?

- Colour rinses
- Coloured setting lotion
- Coloured mousses
- Colour gels
- Colour creams
- Colour sprays
- Colour shampoos

What effect does temporary hair colour have on the hair structure?

- Temporary colour molecules are large and they coat the cuticle/sit on the cuticle layer

What are the key points to remember when working with temporary colour?

- Colour will be removed after one shampoo, but this does depend on the porosity of the hair
- It may not colour the hair evenly
- Short-term fashion effects (i.e. sprays) may rub off on collars and pillows
- You cannot lighten hair with temporary colour
- If hair is porous (usually the ends) the colour will 'take' more vibrantly on these areas, producing uneven results and may last for more than one shampoo

How long does it last?

- One shampoo – although this will depend on the porosity of the client's hair

How long should a temporary colour service take?

- Applying a temporary colour should only take you five minutes

What effect does temporary hair colour have on the hair structure?

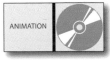

The effect of temporary colour on the hair structure

Colour rinses

These mainly come in two forms:

- Colour concentrates or water rinses
- Prepared, ready to use colour rinses.

These products do not usually contain any added setting or blow-dry lotions.

Coloured setting lotions

These are prepared temporary colour rinses mixed together with setting lotion. Once the client's hair has been shampooed and towel dried comb the hair away from the face. Wearing suitable disposable gloves and a protective apron use one of your hands to shield the face of the client and sprinkle on the lotion/colour rinse through the front hairline, very gently massage the product into the hair. Do not allow the product to sit on the scalp as it may stain. Working back to the nape area, comb or brush the hair through to ensure even distribution.

Coloured mousses

This type of product is based on the same principle as colour setting lotions except they are in a mousse form. They are applied to the hair and do not reqire a development time, they are dried directly into the hair.

Equipment required for a colour mousse application:

- Towel
- Suitable disposable gloves
- Vent brush or comb
- Coloured mousse

STEP BY STEP: APPLICATION OF A COLOUR MOUSSE

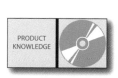

PRODUCT KNOWLEDGE

Colour mousse

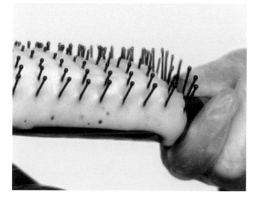

1. Apply mousse to a vent brush for even distribution

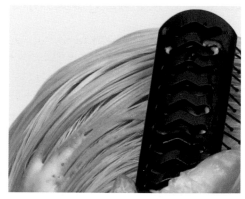

2. Spread mousse from roots to ends

Colour gels mascara and creams

These products are constantly being updated. They are usually found in high fashion, vibrant colours and are applied directly to dry hair.

TIP	
Be careful with some very intense products as they can 'take' on porous hair and you may have difficulty in shampooing them out. In other words, it can last more than one shampoo!	

Colour sprays

Ranges are available from glowing neon orange to pure glitter. They are great for special occasions and the majority will brush out before shampooing.

Colour sprays are applied directly to dry hair; make sure you hold the spray at least 10–12 inches away from the hair when spraying.

TIP	
For temporary colour application plastic capes are not usually necessary, but do place one around the client if the product you are applying stains easily, e.g., reds, mahogany or dark brown.	

TIP	
For semi-permanent and quasi (tone on tone) colours you should always place a plastic cape around the shoulders and secure carefully. Once the semi-permanent and quasi colour has been rinsed off remove and dispose of the plastic cape.	

Colour-enhancing shampoos

These products can help to top up permanent colour by adding colour tone to the hair between the client's salon appointments. It is also great for adding subtle tones ranging from silver to red and copper to natural hair. They are usually applied as the second shampoo and left for a few moments before the final rinse.

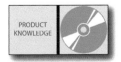

PRODUCT KNOWLEDGE

TIP	
Products may penetrate into the cortex if the hair is very porous. Be careful when using strong tones on porous hair, as it may become more than a one-wash colour.	

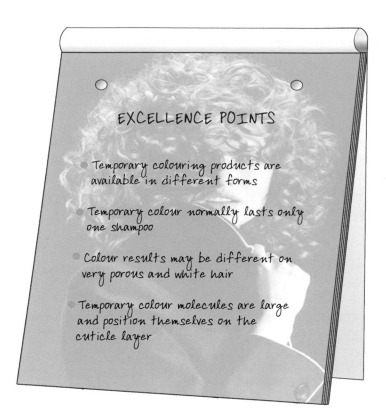

EXCELLENCE POINTS

- Temporary colouring products are available in different forms

- Temporary colour normally lasts only one shampoo

- Colour results may be different on very porous and white hair

- Temporary colour molecules are large and position themselves on the cuticle layer

SEMI-PERMANENT COLOUR

Semi-permanent colours are fantastic versatile products that give the hairdresser flexibility when recommending colour services to clients. Because these products only last 6–8 shampoos, you can use them on 'colour shy' clients as an introduction to colour (a good selling point would be to promote semi-permanents as colouring conditioners, as these products contain high quality conditioning ingredients that always give fantastic shine as well as lovely colour tone). Another great way to use semi-permanent colours is on your existing permanent colour clientele as colour top ups, especially the fashion reds and coppers. Booking these clients between their permanent colour appointments will keep the colour fresh and the hair in good condition.

A selection of semi-permanent colour products

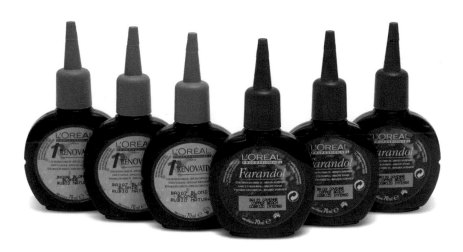

Why would we use a semi-permanent colour product on a client's hair?

- To refresh permanent colour, perfect for in-between colour appointments
- Can be used for colour corrective work (pre-pigmentation)
- Tone pre-lightened hair
- Great for a colour/conditioning treatment. These products contain no ammonia and do not require hydrogen peroxide, they are perfect to give hair shine and vitality
- Does not leave a regrowth
- Colour will wash out approximately 6–8 shampoos, this will depend on the porosity of the hair
- To add tone to white hair – this will create a diffused blending by colouring white hair which creates a very natural effect
- Can provide an alternative colour choice for clients who are allergic/sensitive to permanent dyes
- It will last longer than a temporary colour
- Vibrant 'crazy colours' are available for high street fashion results on lighter depths or pre-lightened hair

What are the key points to remember when working with semi-permanent colour?

- It lasts 6–8 shampoos
- It is ideal for clients who are new to colour or 'colour shy' as there is no long-term commitment.
- If hair is porous (usually the ends) the colour may take more vibrantly on these areas, producing uneven results and lasting more than 6–8 shampoos
- Will only colour from 25–60 per cent on white hair according to which semi-permanent product you are using. Always refer to the manufacturer's instructions
- If used as part of a colour corrective procedure it will need to be reapplied after 6–8 shampoos to maintain the colour

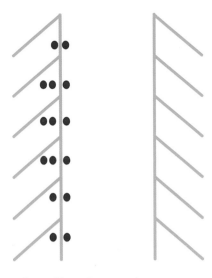

What effect does semi-permanent hair colour have on the hair structure?

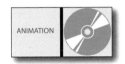

The effect of semi-permanent hair colour on the hair structure

What different types are there?

- Gel
- Mousse
- Liquid
- Cream

How long does it last?

- 6–8 shampoos
- Semi-permanent colour will be reduced by general wear and tear and repeated shampooing

What effect does semi-permanent hair colour have on the hair structure?

- Large molecules will coat and lie on the cuticle, small molecules will lie on the cortex
- Semi-permanent colour contains a mix of large and small molecules

How long should a semi-permanent colour service take?

- Application plus development times – remember this will vary depending on the manufacturer's instructions

STEP BY STEP: APPLICATION OF A SEMI-PERMANENT COLOUR

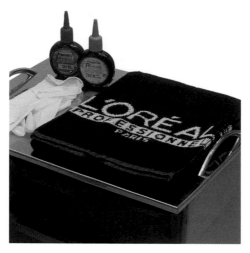

1. Equipment required for colour application

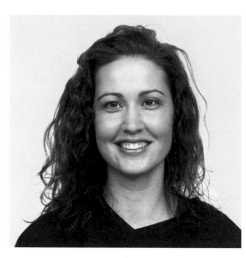

2. Before colour application

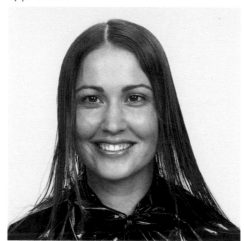

3. Shampoo the hair

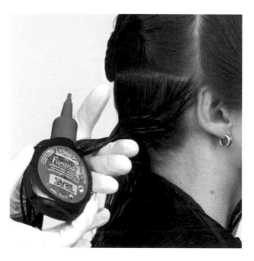

4. Apply the product directly from the bottle

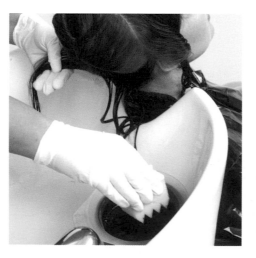

5. Alternatively, use a sponge to make the application

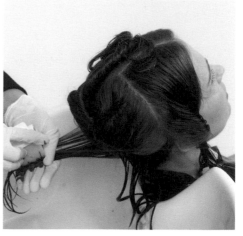

6. Apply evenly through the hair, from root to points

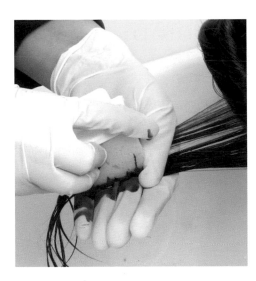

7. Continue application

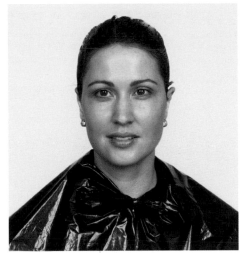

8. Leave for full development time

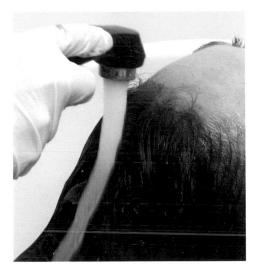

9. Rinse thoroughly until water runs clear

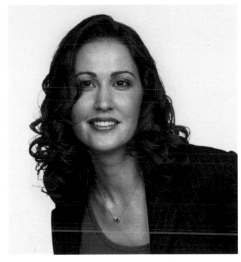

10. Final result

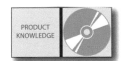

PRODUCT KNOWLEDGE

Semi-permanent: gel, liquid and cream

Gel, liquid and cream

Always read the manufacturer's instructions accompanying the product that you are using. Shampoo and towel dry the hair and make sure your client is properly gowned, protected and comfortable, then section the hair into four sections – centre of forehead through to centre of nape and ear to ear. Think of a hot cross bun! Using a tint brush apply from roots to ends ensuring all hair has been covered. You can also apply semi-permanent colour straight from the bottle or with a tint bowl and a clean sponge. The manufacturer's instructions should give guidance as to the best application method.

HEALTH AND SAFETY ➕

Always make sure you protect yourself and your client when applying a semi-permanent colour.

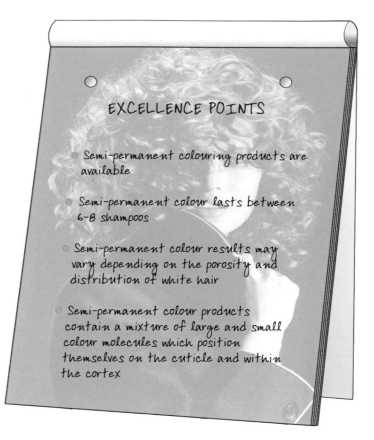

EXCELLENCE POINTS

- Semi-permanent colouring products are available

- Semi-permanent colour lasts between 6-8 shampoos

- Semi-permanent colour results may vary depending on the porosity and distribution of white hair

- Semi-permanent colour products contain a mixture of large and small colour molecules which position themselves on the cuticle and within the cortex

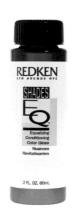

QUASI (TONE ON TONE) COLOUR

Quasi or tone on tone products are very versatile for today's hairdressers. They can be used for colour correction techniques, combination techniques such as foils with the quasi (tone on tone) applied between the packets to get a really beautiful result. They are also good for clients with varying amounts of white hair to blend and diffuse with the existing natural depth to give shine and vitality.

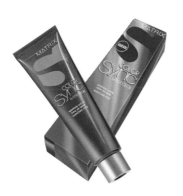

Why would we use a quasi (tone on tone) colour on a client's hair?

- Clients who have used a semi-permanent but would like the effect to last longer
- It is a good introduction for first time colour clients
- To add depth
- To add tone
- These products can colour higher percentages of white hair (please refer to individual manufacturer's instructions for guidance)
- To produce fashion effects
- To refresh faded colour between permanent colour appointments
- Can be used in colour correction procedures
- To be applied during fashion techniques i.e. between Easi Meche wraps or foils to colour the remaining hair

What are the key points to remember when working with quasi (tone on tone) colour?

- This could produce a demarcation (regrowth) line when darker or more vibrant tones are used
- It will only add depth and tone
- It cannot lighten hair colour

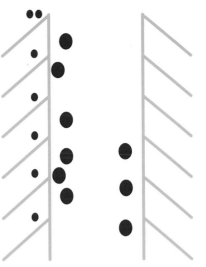

What effect does quasi (tone on tone) hair colour have on the hair structure?

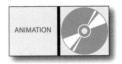

The effect of quasi (tone on tone) hair colour on the hair structure

What different types are there?

- Creams
- Gel

How long does it last?

- Many shampoos, depending on the condition of the hair
- This product is designed to fade over time

What effect does quasi (tone on tone) hair colour have on the hair structure?

- Deposit only, they have a mix of small and medium colour molecules
- The medium molecules penetrate into the cortex
- The small molecules will penetrate and coat the cuticle and lie in the cortex

How long should a quasi (tone on tone) colour service take?

- Application time plus development time, depending on the manufacturer's instructions

---

TIP

Quasi (tone on tone) products evolved because of demand from the hairdressing industry. Hairdressers and clients were looking for a result between semi and permanent colour. Manufacturers developed quasi (tone on tone) technology creating ready made shades that hairdressers can rely on.

STEP BY STEP: APPLICATION OF A QUASI (TONE ON TONE) COLOUR

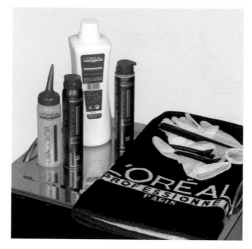

1. Equipment required for application

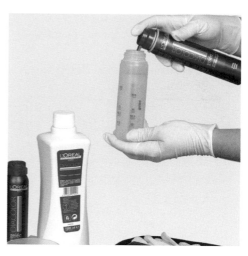

2. Mix product as directed

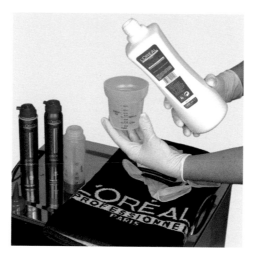

3. Measure required oxidant

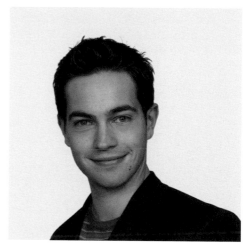

4. Before colour application

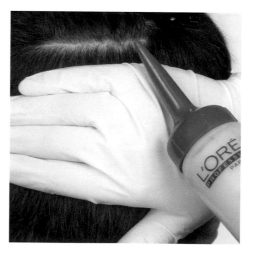

5. Section the hair to start application

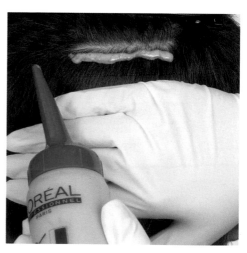

6. Begin application at root area

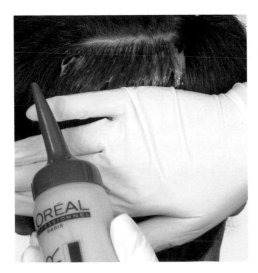

7. Spread evenly through hair

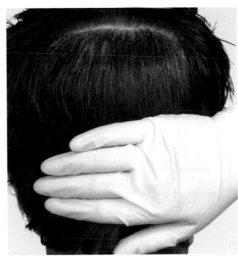

8. Continue with application

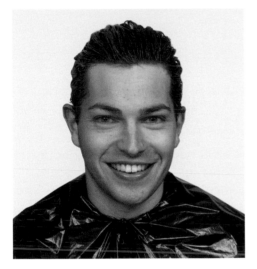

9. Leave for full development time

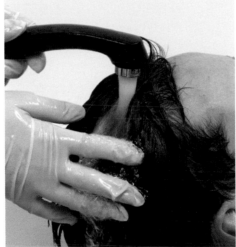

10. Add water to emulsify and rinse

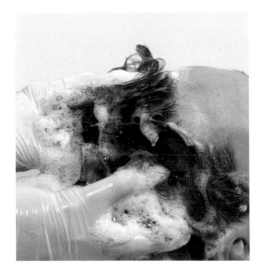

11. Shampoo gently

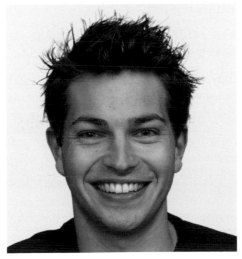

12. Final result

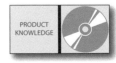

PRODUCT KNOWLEDGE

Quasi (tone on tone) colour

TIP ✔

Always express the importance of styling products.

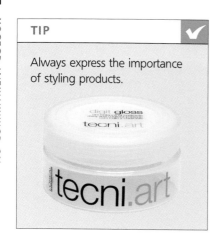

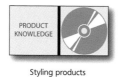

PRODUCT KNOWLEDGE

Styling products

HEALTH AND SAFETY ✚

Some clients may be sensitive to quasi (tone on tone) products, so make sure that they have a skin allergy test 48 hours prior to the colour service.

TIP ✔

Quasi (tone on tone) colours last for many shampoos depending on the frequency of shampooing. For example: a client who washes their hair every day will see the intensity of their colour reduce quicker than a client who only washes their hair twice a week.

TIP ✔

To change a quasi (tone on tone) colour, depending on the desired shade, you may need to use colour correction techniques. See Chapter Four.

ORGANIC HENNA – NATURAL COLOUR

Henna is the oldest recorded colour that is still being used even today. As with fashion, colour trends and products come and go but organic henna still retains its place within the market. It is enjoying a small revival now and is being marketed in high street health and beauty shops. Organic henna will always have an appeal to some people who want to colour their hair but wish to use natural products.

Henna comes from the plant *Lawsonia inermis* and the leaves are chopped and ground into fine powder.

Red henna is the basic *Lawsonia* powder and the most pure form, producing reddish tones.

Neutral henna or **senna** (*Cassia oborate*) tends to stain in the golden blonde range.

Black henna or **indigo** (*Indigotera tinctoria*) or in some cases woad (*Isatis tinctoria*) is a strictly botanical product. When mixed, it has a green appearance and an unpleasant smell.

Blonde, brown, auburn, mahogany and other shades of henna are mixes of zizphus, indigo and true henna, often with plant materials such as hibiscus and black walnut to enhance the different tones available.

You mix the powder into a thick paste with hot water and apply onto shampooed and towel dried hair. For best results the paste needs to develop for up to five hours.

In some cases, you can use heat to speed the process up: make sure you wrap the client's head in cling film or a plastic cap to retain the moisture in the henna paste. Otherwise, it will dry and flake away from the hair shaft.

Camomile is produced from the camomile plant and develops a golden yellow tone to already blonde hair. It will have no effect on darker bases of hair. Camomile is mainly formulated within shampoo, making it very easy to apply.

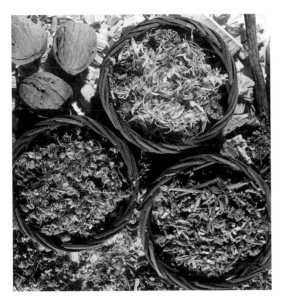
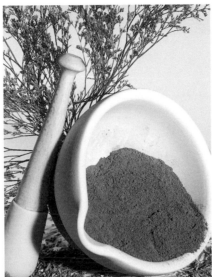

A selection of organic hair colour

HEALTH AND SAFETY

It can be a very messy business, so be prepared. Henna will stain not only the client's hair but everything it touches: be careful!

TIP

When colouring with organic henna, the end result will be a lot brighter on porous and white hair.

Why would we use organic colour on a client's hair?

- Organic/natural colours can be an alternative for clients who are allergic to oxidation/permanent colours
- Good for clients who do not like chemicals on their hair

What are the limitations of organic/natural colour?

- It can produce a regrowth with darker shades
- It will only add tone
- It cannot lighten hair
- May not be compatible with an oxidation process

What are the key points to remember when working with organic colour?

- The application and development of these products is very time-consuming
- The shade range is limited
- Results could be very vibrant and artificial-looking on white hair
- It will stain all porous surfaces

What different types are there?

- Organic henna
- Camomile

How long does it last?

- Organic henna will fade but is permanent, so can only be removed by cutting
- Camomile will fade over several shampoos

What effect does organic colour have on the hair structure?

- It coats the hair shaft and seals the cuticle

How long should an organic colour service take?

- Several hours – refer to the manufacturer's instructions

TIP	
Be aware of your client's comfort throughout the colouring service and ensure they are adequately protected. If the towels get damp replace them with fresh dry ones.	

TIP	
If possible always try to turn the client's collar inside out before placing the towel around the shoulders, as this will give the client extra protection against any spills or colour run.	

READING AND FOLLOWING THE MANUFACTURER'S INSTRUCTIONS

When using any colouring product *always* make sure you read the manufacturer's instructions. Even if you are familiar with a particular procedure whilst carrying out a colouring service, manufacturers are continually updating and improving their products and in turn changing the instructions, so make sure you update your knowledge by being aware of any changes.

CLIENT PROTECTION AND SAFETY

After consultation always gown your client, remembering to cover and protect the customer's clothes. Place one towel around the shoulders, tucking the towel into the collar if possible. Secure towel at the front with a butterfly clip to stop the towel from falling off the client midway through the service.

HEALTH AND SAFETY	

Colouring precautions
When colouring hair always carry out necessary hair tests to protect the client and yourself. Carefully read and follow the manufacturer's instructions and ensure that when removing colouring products you leave no residue on the hair or scalp.

YOUR PERSONAL PROTECTION AND SAFETY

When applying any colouring product always be prepared with suitable disposable gloves and protective apron. This will ensure that you keep clean and tidy while undertaking the colouring service on your client's hair and promotes a professional image and your client's confidence in your ability as a hairdresser.

Prepare your workstation

When you prepare for the day ahead you need to set out equipment that you are going to need within easy reach on your workstation. This will make you more efficient while you are working which promotes a professional image and creates confidence and trust in your client.

TIP	

It is very important that you take care of your personal hygiene to minimise offence to clients and colleagues. It will also reduce the risk of cross-infection and cross-infestation (see Chapter 5).

ACTIVITY	

Write a salon policy on how you protect yourself and your client's clothing during colouring services. Include details of how you would protect a client's skin and what tests could be carried out during consultation.

TIP

Electrical equipment
When using electrical equipment always do a visual check to see if there could be any faults. Look for any loose wires or plugs – this will minimise the risk of harm that you could do to yourself and to others – and ensure that the equipment is in good working order.

TIP

Always leave your work area clean and tidy to minimise the risk of cross-infection, reduce hazards and to maintain a professional image.

Heat

Temperature is very important to the development of technical colour products as it can speed up or slow down the processing time therefore a heat source such as an accelerator may be used with some products.

It is important to refer to each product's individual guidelines to check if it is appropriate to use heat and what changes it will make to the development time. Remember that not all products react well to heat.

Before using any electrical equipment make sure it has been safety checked and is in good working order to minimize the risk of any harm to yourself and others.

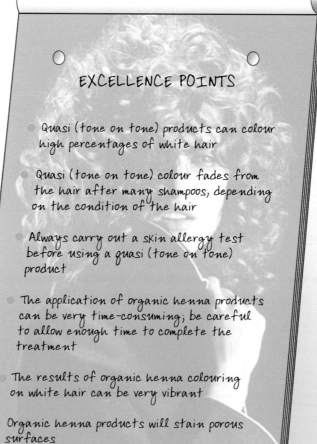

EXCELLENCE POINTS

- Quasi (tone on tone) products can colour high percentages of white hair

- Quasi (tone on tone) colour fades from the hair after many shampoos, depending on the condition of the hair

- Always carry out a skin allergy test before using a quasi (tone on tone) product

- The application of organic henna products can be very time-consuming; be careful to allow enough time to complete the treatment

- The results of organic henna colouring on white hair can be very vibrant

- Organic henna products will stain porous surfaces

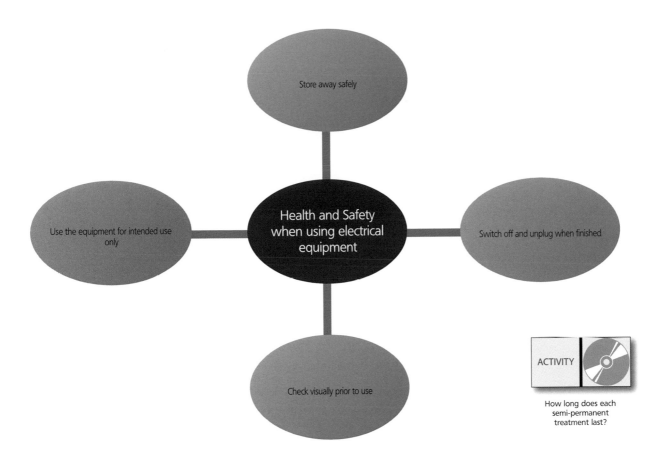

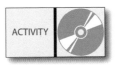

ACTIVITY

How long does each semi-permanent treatment last?

Assessment of knowledge and understanding

Test yourself on the content of this chapter by answering these questions. This will help you to prepare for your Essential knowledge/Written test.

1   What are the different types of protective equipment available? Explain why it is important to use personal protective equipment.

2   Why is it important to position your colouring tools and equipment so that they are easier for you to use?

3   What are the safety considerations that you must carry out when you are colouring hair?

4   Give two reasons why work areas should be kept and left clean and tidy.

5   Why is it essential to have good personal hygiene?

6   Why should you always check electrical equipment before you use it?

7   Give two reasons for the importance of following manufacturer's instructions when using colouring products.

8   Draw and describe three line diagrams demonstrating how temporary, semi-permanent and quasi-permanent (tone on tone) colours affect the hair structure, including how long each colour product lasts.

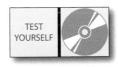

ACTIVITY

Wordsearch

TEST YOURSELF

Testing and essential knowledge

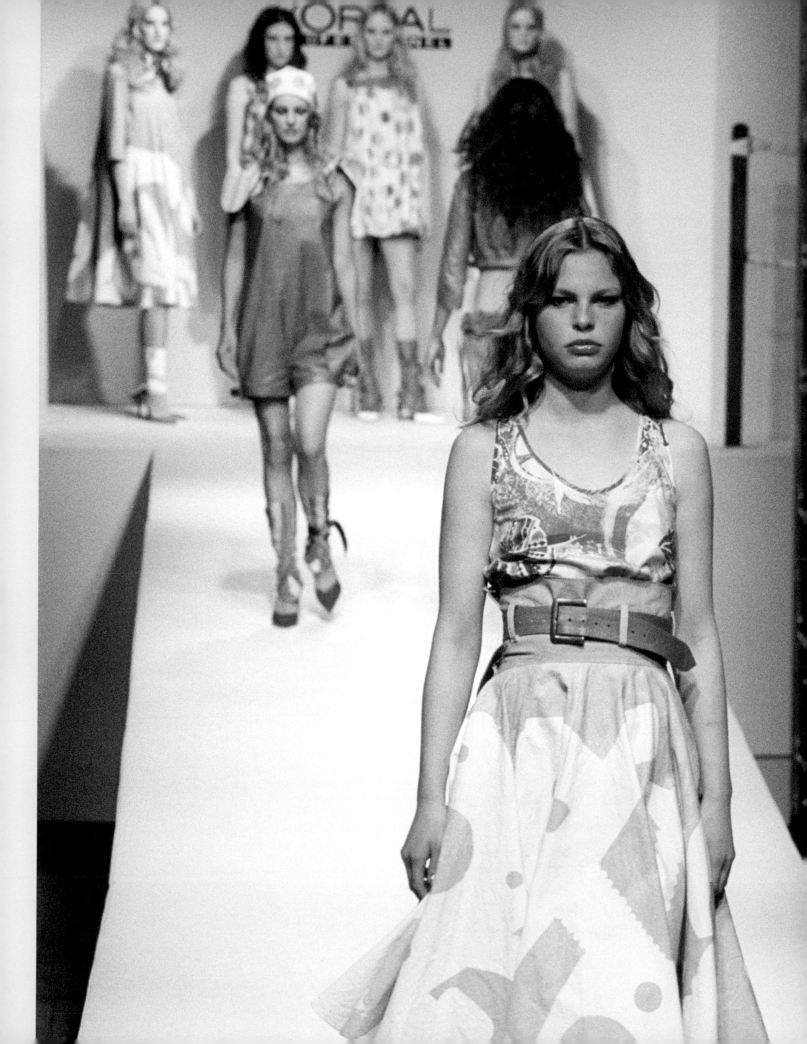

Commit to colour

Cut and colour work hand in hand to create the total individual look.

Jo O'Neill, International Technical Director, Toni & Guy

If you're going out to a party, you probably don't wear the same clothes as you would for walking the dog. For different occasions, we want to create a specific image or look. We use make-up, clothes, jewellery or accessories. They all affect the end result, and it's the same with colour.

As a colourist, it's not just the different colours you use but *how* you use them. How you place colour can affect the shape of a haircut, highlight different shades, intensify or blend.

Now that colour is so much a part of how we look, it's more important than ever to understand your products and how to use them.

Jo O'Neill from Toni & Guy says

"To be a good colourist, you must be precise in your technique and work with patience. To be a great colourist, you need to foresee the end result, use your technique to enhance the shape of the cut, and have an extensive knowledge of your products."

With so many new products, innovative techniques and styles changing all the time, you need to be aware, educated, inspired and updated throughout your career. Stay creative, keep learning.

chapter 3

COMMIT TO COLOUR

In this chapter you will learn how to change hair colour using permanent colouring and pre-lightening products. You will gain an understanding of global colouring (full head), regrowth application and highlight and lowlight effects. In *commit to colour*, we will consider:

- **Permanent colour**
- **How does permanent colour work within the hair structure?**
- **Skin allergy testing**
- **The colour wheel**
- **Primary and secondary tones**
- **International Colour Code (ICC) or Numbering system**
- **Shade charts**
- **White hair**
- **Pre-softening**
- **How to achieve the correct shade according to the client's natural hair colour**
- **Permanent colour application techniques**
- **Identifying the hair's artificial colour**
- **Refreshing the lengths and ends when permanently colouring the hair**
- **Using heat during permanent colouring services**
- **Permanent colour removal**
- **Points to remember when carrying out a colouring service**
- **The effects natural and artificial light can have on permanent colour**
- **Bleaching (pre-lightening) hair**
- **Bleaching (pre-lightening) application techniques**
- **Trouble shooting: common colouring problems and solutions**

H30 Colour hair using a variety of techniques

PERMANENT COLOUR

Permanent colours are produced in a wide variety of tones and shades. They can colour white and natural hair to create a wide range of natural, fashion and fantasy effects.

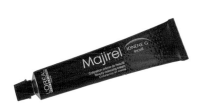

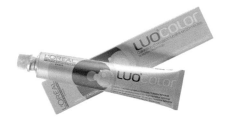

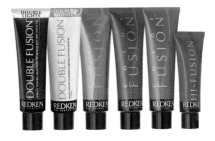

A selection of permanent colour products

How does permanent colour work?

Hydrogen peroxide of different strengths and in varying quantities is mixed with the permanent colour; this allows the resulting oxidation tint to produce different results.

What's in a tube of oxidation tint?

- Support – all oxidation colour products come in the form of cream, liquid or gel. This is the 'support' or main body of the tint. They come in tubes, cans or bottles.
- Ammonia – releases oxygen from the oxidant (which is mixed with the tint to activate it). This swells the hair to enable the colour to penetrate the cuticle.
- Colour precursors – these are colourless molecules, which, through the oxidation process, are transformed into coloured molecules of linear shape (traditional colourants) or multidimensional shape molecules (high tenacity colourants).
- Antioxidant – this preserves the formula in the tube and extends the shelf life of the colour for up to three years.
- Cosmetic agents – these are added to the oxidation tint to protect the hair during and after the colour process to ensure a durable colour result.

How do these components work together?

Ammonia swells the hair to facilitate the penetration of the colour product. At the same time it acts on the oxidant, freeing the oxygen, enabling it to oxidise which lightens the hair pigments. At the same time the oxygen acts on the colour precursors, transforming them during the development time into colour molecules.

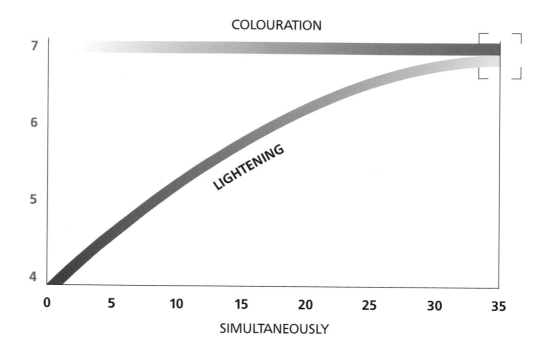

COLOURATION

LIGHTENING

SIMULTANEOUSLY

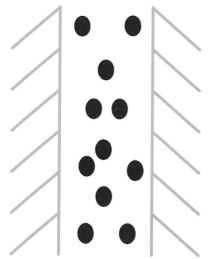

How does permanent hair colour work within the hair structure?

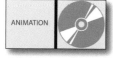

ANIMATION

Effect of permanent colour on the hair structure

How does permanent hair colour work within the hair structure?

Hydrogen peroxide (H_2O_2) helps to swell the hair shaft (cuticle) and oxidises the hair's natural pigments. This enables the small molecules of artificial pigment to join together retaining the colour permanently within the cortex: this process is called polymerisation. Because different product companies have different levels of ammonia and para dyes contained within their tubes of colour, different strengths of hydrogen peroxide may be needed to produce different results.

For example

- The higher the percentage or volume strength of oxidant (hydrogen peroxide), the more oxygen is available.
- The more oxygen that is released into the hair, the higher the degree of colour lift that can be obtained.
- If the required result is to remain the same depth or darker, less oxygen is needed and the percentage or volume strength of hydrogen peroxide would be lower.

TIP	

Always refer to the manufacturer's instructions when using permanent colouring products as some products use a specific developer in order to achieve a range of colour effects, depending on the colour selection.

What is the lightening power of a permanent tint?

You can only lighten hair to a certain degree with permanent colour; this will depend on the existing natural depth and the tone of the client's hair. If your client has a warm tone reflecting within their hair colour, it could affect the amount of lighting that you wish to achieve; warm tones in the cortex of the hair indicate that it contains a lot of diffuse pigment (pheomelanin), which can be more resistant to achieving your target shade. (See How to achieve the correct target shade according to the client's natural colour, p. 62). In addition, the percentage/volume of peroxide that you would be using will dictate the levels of lightening that you will achieve. All permanent colours come with full instructions on the degree of lightening that their products can achieve, but always refer to your manufacturer's instructions for specific guidelines.

Oxidation colour works on two principles; it simultaneously lightens and colours.

The table below is a guide to the level of lightening a permanent colour can achieve when colouring hair.

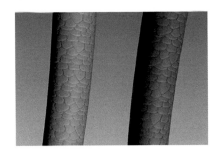

Natural colour pigment

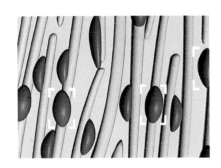

Granular (melanin) pigment

Hydrogen peroxide strength

Percentage	Volume	*The effect it has on the hair*	
6	20 vol	● Coverage of white hair	● Below a base 4
		● Darken the hair	● Hair will lighten 1 level
		● Colouring to the same depth as the client's hair	
		● Lighten the hair one level	
		● Lighten the hair two levels	
9	30 vol	● Lighten the hair three levels	● Below a base 4
			● Hair will lighten 2 levels
12	40 vol	● Lighten the hair up to four levels	

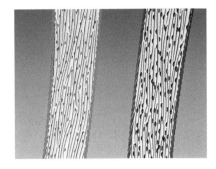

Granular (melanin) pigment

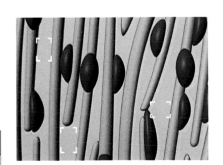

Diffused (pheamelanin) pigment

TIP ✔

Development times
It is important that oxidation colours are allowed to develop correctly. If you remove the colour from the hair before it has developed correctly the following will occur:

● The expected lightening will not be obtained

● The undercoat will be too warm; this will dominate the target shade

● The colour molecules would not be allowed to develop fully, resulting in a wishy-washy tone

● The colour will fade quickly.

L'Oréal Professionnel Levels of
Lighting Chart

Depth No.	Depth Name	Pigment	Level of lightening
10	Lightest Blonde		Very Pale Yellow
9	Very light Blonde		Pale Yellow
8	Light Blonde		Yellow
7	Blonde		Yellow Orange
6	Dark Blonde		Orange
5	Light Brown		Orange Red
4	Brown		Red
3	Dark Brown		Red
2	Darkest Brown		Red
1	Black		Red

The levels of lightening chart above can be used by colourists as a guide to estimate the underlying tones of the natural pigment when working with permanent colour. Each depth of colour has a corresponding undercoat, for example: 7 Blonde – yellow orange.

Use the chart to calculate if the hair's underlying tones will be complimentary for your chosen shade.

Case study

Look at each level of lightening/undercoat and how this corresponds to each separate colour depth of hair.

For example

1 Client A has a natural base of 5 – Light brown
   She wants to be two levels lighter
   The result will be Blonde – 7 with a yellow/orange undercoat

2 Client B has a natural base of 6 – Dark blonde
   She wants to be three levels lighter
   The result will be Very light blonde – 9 with a pale yellow undercoat

3 Client C has a natural base of 5 – Light brown
   She wants to be two shades darker
   The result will be Dark brown – 3 with a yellow orange undercoat.
   This is because Client C has become artificially two shades darker but her natural undercoat has still lightened.

Care of hydrogen peroxide (oxidant)

Always store hydrogen peroxide in a cool dark cupboard, and *always* screw the cap back on to the bottle as soon as you have measured the required amount; this will retain the maximum strength of the hydrogen peroxide. If the bottle is left open to the atmosphere, it is dangerous; if it is spilt the hydrogen peroxide will degrade and break down into a lesser volume (percentage). This will give you an unreliable result with future colouring services when using that particular bottle (there will be less volume as O_2 – oxygen – is released as gas, resulting in a diluted effect).

$$*H_2O_2 \longrightarrow H_2O + O_2$$

(Hydrogen peroxide) will break down to (water) + (oxygen)

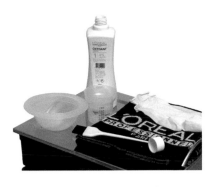

Never leave the cap off when working with hydrogen peroxide

TIP ✔

Good quality oxidants will contain stabilising agents to help protect against destabilisation.

TIP ✔

This is an example of how you would dilute different strengths of hydrogen peroxide (**you can only dilute liquid peroxide** to get an accurate result). In the dilution process of hydrogen peroxide you can use a hydrometer or peroxometer to test the strength of the peroxide that you have and the strength of the peroxide once you have diluted it.

Hydrogen peroxide that you have	Hydrogen peroxide that you want to dilute it to	Answer
9%	6%	1:2 One part water, two parts hydrogen peroxide
12%	6%	1:1 One part water, one part hydrogen peroxide
18%	9%	1:1 One part water, one part hydrogen peroxide

Note: Manufacturers today mass-produce oxidants in the required volume strengths for safe use.

ACTIVITY

Diluting hydrogen peroxide

ACTIVITY

Testing of essential knowledge on oxidant strengths

HEALTH AND SAFETY ✚

COSHH (Control of Substances Hazardous to Heath Regulations)

Remember always store, handle, use and dispose of colouring products according to salon policy, manufacturers' instructions and local by-laws.

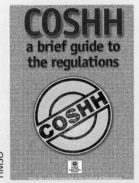

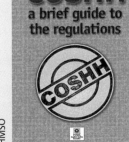

COSHH
a brief guide to the regulations

HMSO

POINTS TO REMEMBER WHEN PREPARING FOR A PERMANENT COLOUR SERVICE

Make sure your client has had a skin allergy test 48 hours before the colour application. Most manufacturers recommend that you perform a skin allergy test before every permanent and quasi (tone on tone) colour service. Always check the manufacturers' guidelines.

TIP
Client care Even if your client has had the same colour for a long time always do a full consultation. Never be complacent with your regular colour clients as this could lead to loss of business.

How to carry out a skin allergy test

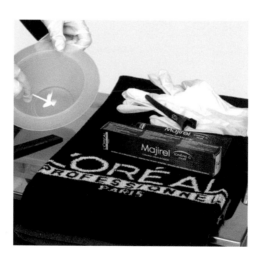
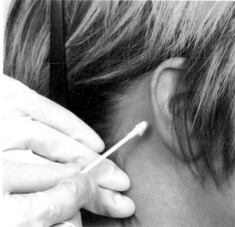

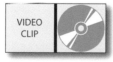

Skin allergy testing

Remove the client's earrings. Behind the ear and using a cotton-bud, apply a little of the unmixed colourant product sufficient to cover 1cm^2. Re-apply 2 or 3 times allowing it to dry between each application. Leave for 48 hours without washing, covering or touching.

If during the 48 hours after the test you or your client notices any abnormal reaction such as intense redness, itching or swelling in or around the test area DO NOT APPLY THE COLOURANT. Recommend that your client seeks medical advice before any colour applications are made.

THE IMPORTANCE OF READING AND UNDERSTANDING THE MANUFACTURER'S INSTRUCTIONS AND RECOMMENDATIONS

When measuring and mixing colouring and lightening products it is *essential* to follow the manufacturer's instructions to ensure that the correct colour result is attained and to avoid damage to the hair and scalp. When taking medication you would always read the instructions on the side of the bottle, because you are aware of their importance and do not want to take the wrong dosage. Manufacturers' instructions are just as important when carrying out a colour service. Colouring products change all the time due to the high level of competition within the hairdressing industry and the instructions can change so *always check to make sure*.

Health and Safety checklist when colouring and bleaching (pre-lightening) hair

- You must always carry out the necessary hair and skin allergy tests (see Chapter 6)
- Always use clean protective materials for you and your clients
- Always wear suitable disposable gloves and aprons (Personal Protective Equipment Act, see Chapter 6)
- Always sterilise your tools and equipment
- Make sure the client is comfortable and in the correct position for you to be able to work efficiently, minimising fatigue and the risk of injury. The client should be seated with their back against the chair to reduce slouching, enabling the hairdresser to carry out the colouring service correctly. The hairdresser should always stand with their feet slightly apart to evenly distribute their weight. Too much stretching and bending could lead to long-term personal injury
- Always read and follow the manufacturer's instructions
- Always keep your work area clean and tidy throughout the service
- Dispose of waste according to COSHH regulations and local by-laws, all unused products should be diluted and rinsed away (refer to Chapter 6)
- Ensure thorough and careful removal of colouring and bleaching (pre-lightening) products and materials
- Supervise colleagues who assist in the colour and bleaching (pre-lightening) process.

THE PRINCIPLES OF OXIDATION COLOURING – THE COLOUR WHEEL

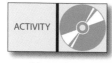

ACTIVITY

Primary colours

To understand the principles of oxidation colouring, you need to understand the colour wheel and why it is especially important when we talk about:

- Primary and secondary colours
- Neutralisation.

Primary and secondary tones

The colour wheel consists of primary and secondary colours. Primary colours are blue, red and yellow; secondary colours are green, purple and orange.

The colour wheel

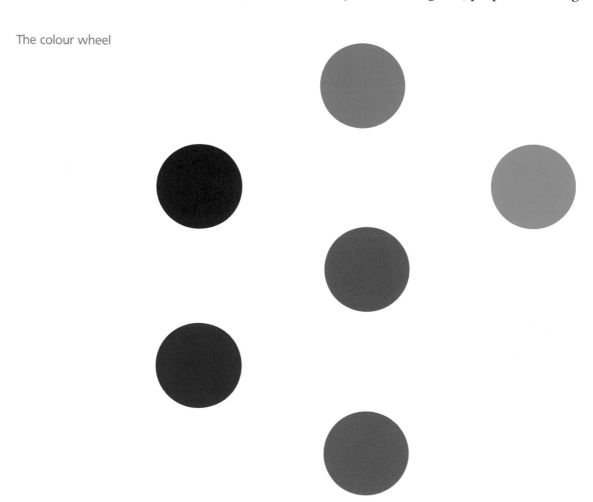

Secondary colours are created by mixing different combinations of primary colours, following the colour circle clockwise:

- Mix red and yellow to produce orange
- Mix yellow and blue to produce green
- Mix blue and red to produce purple.

THE INTERNATIONAL COLOUR CODE (ICC) OR NUMBERING SYSTEM

The ICC is a generic system for the hairdressing industry around the world to guide hairdressers through the products of different colouring companies. It creates a structure to which manufacturers of permanent colouring products can adhere. However, although almost all of these rules are followed by the different companies, there are certain differences between manufacturers. For example the numbers given to tones – red for example – could differ between different product ranges, so always get to know the shade chart that you work with. It is an interesting exercise to compare the differences between companies.

- The depth of colour refers to how light or dark the colour and is the first number recorded. Think of a scale of black to very light blonde hair.

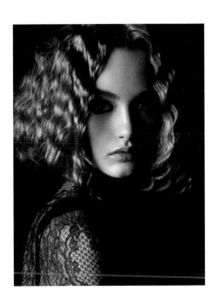

Depths of hair colours

10 Lightest blonde

9 Very light blonde

8 Light blonde

7 Blonde

6 Dark blonde

5 Light brown

4 Brown

3 Dark brown

2 Darkest brown

1 Black

TIP

A quick way to assess your client's hair colour.

First, is the client's hair colour black, brown or blonde? Once you have established that, ask yourself is it dark, medium or light? Check your results with the shade chart.

ACTIVITY

Tones
Draw your own colour wheel, label it and colour it in with appropriate coloured pencils. Then look at all the different tones across a shade chart. Can you match the tones to the colour wheel?

Tones

● The tone is the colour that you see and is the number recorded after the depth. Tones range from warm shades such as gold, copper, red to cool shades such as mauve and various ash shades.
(See example below of L'Oréal Professionnel's numbering system).

In some cases, using a shade chart with your colour client is a valuable tool when deciding together the colour that is to be used. The first number after the comma represents the primary tone. The second number represents the secondary tone.

● Blue = ,1 represents ash

● Purple = ,2 represents mauve ash iridescent

● Yellow = ,3 represents gold

● Orange = ,4 represents copper

● Red + purple = ,5 represents mahogany

● Red = ,6 represents red

● Green = ,7 represents metallic

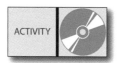

ACTIVITY

Tones and numbering
system

blue ash	mauve ash (iridescent)	gold	copper	mahogany	red	metallic
,1	,2	,3	,4	,5	,6	,7

10

9

8

7

6

5

4

3

2

1

4 4 5

The depth-or how light or dark the hair

Primary tone

Secondary tone

Warm and cool tones

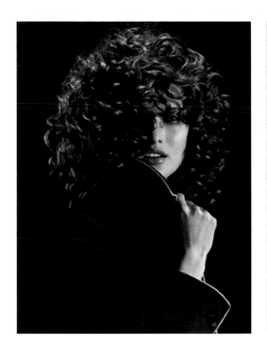

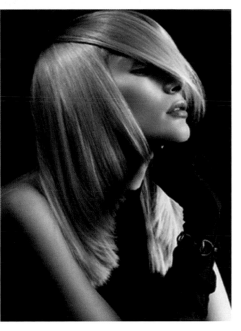

L'Oréal Professionnel tones fit into two sectors:

1 Cool tones = 1–blue, 2–mauve ash iridescent and 5–mahogany: these will absorb light and often appear one shade darker

2 Warm tones = 3–gold, 4–copper, 5–mahogany and 6-red: these will reflect light and appear one shade lighter.

Mahogany contains both warm and cool tones so can be classed as either warm or cool; the classification would be determined by the secondary tone.

Case study

For example:

Your client has Majirel 5.52
on her hair =   Depth of 5 Light brown
                                 Primary tone .5 = Mahogany (cool)
                                 Secondary tone .2 = Ash iridescent (cool)

Is this a warm or cool mahogany?

Your client has Majirel 4.56
on her hair =   Depth of 4 Brown
                                 Primary tone .5 = Mahogany (cool)
                                 Secondary tone .6 = Red (warm)

Is this a warm or cool mahogany?

Neutralisation

The colour wheel is used during colour services for neutralisation as the opposite colours on the circle will counteract unwanted natural tones. For example:

- Green tones will neutralise unwanted red
- Blue tones will neutralise unwanted orange
- Purple tones will neutralise unwanted yellow

Tone and numbering system

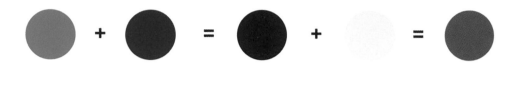

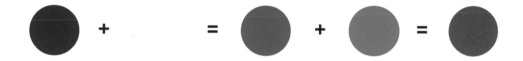

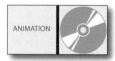

ANIMATION

Complementary colours and
neutralisation summary

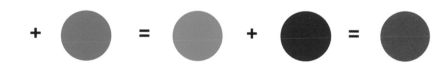

TIP	

Shade chart
The colours of the wheel become numbers that we as hairdressers relate to and use but it will mean nothing to your client. When referring to the tones with your client use the names in the shade chart as opposed to the numbers.

TIP	

When adding three primary colours together, the resulting colour will be a neutral shade according to the rules of neutralisation.

EXCELLENCE POINTS

- The colour wheel can be used to understand neutralisation

- Depth refers to how light or dark the colour is

- Tone refers to how warm or cool the colour is

- Shade charts can be used as valuable visual aids

- The International Colour Code (ICC) represents the generic code to understand the composition of a tint

- The primary tone is the strongest tone, the secondary tone is the weakest

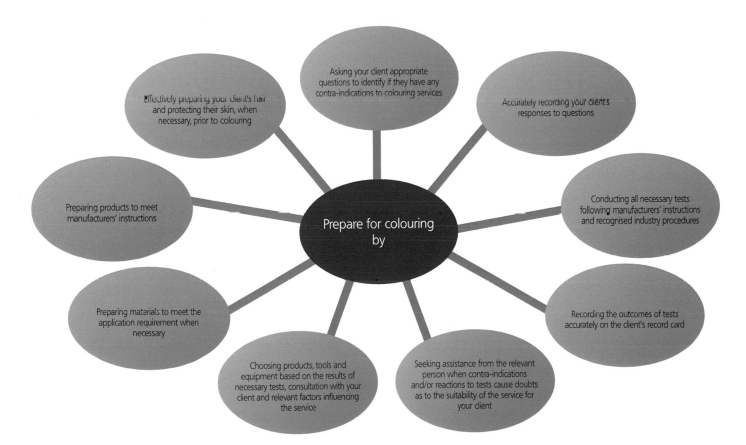

Prepare for colouring by

- Asking your client appropriate questions to identify if they have any contra-indications to colouring services

- Effectively preparing your client's hair and protecting their skin, when necessary, prior to colouring

- Accurately recording your clients responses to questions

- Preparing products to meet manufacturers' instructions

- Conducting all necessary tests following manufacturers' instructions and recognised industry procedures

- Preparing materials to meet the application requirement when necessary

- Recording the outcomes of tests accurately on the client's record card

- Choosing products, tools and equipment based on the results of necessary tests, consultation with your client and relevant factors influencing the service

- Seeking assistance from the relevant person when contra-indications and/or reactions to tests cause doubts as to the suitability of the service for your client

White hair

White hair is normally a different texture to natural pigmented hair, and this can make it resistant to permanent colour. Hair is white because the melanocytes stop making the pigment melanin and the hair produced is actually colourless. Why white hair appears is still unknown. We know that the ageing process is a factor and that any sudden stressful situation, such as suffering grief from losing a loved one, can cause white hair to appear. However, scientists still do not have a clear explanation of why the melanocytes stop producing melanin.

When white hair starts to appear we as hairdressers need to know how to give advice and guidance to achieve the client's needs and expectations.

There are several options:

- To colour the first signs of white hair (up to 60 per cent), with no commitment direct colour application using semi-permanent colourants; this will give a natural look that restores natural depth and tone. This will blend the white hair as opposed to covering it, and washes out over 6–8 shampoos leaving no regrowth.

- To colour the first signs of white hair (up to 50 per cent) with durability. Use a quasi (tone on tone) colour product but remember that this leaves a regrowth and fades gradually over many shampoos. Use natural shades that will blend in the white hair.

- To cover 100 per cent of white hair, use permanent colour products.

Manufacturers' instructions will indicate how to produce the best results on white hair. When choosing your target shade bear in mind that you have to add depth and tone to white hair, because there is no pigment present. Therefore, you need to make sure you are putting enough colour molecules back into the cortex to establish the new depth and tone. The more white hair that is present, the brighter any warm tones such as red and copper will show up, so be cautious if you are using warm tones on a high percentage of white hair. Shades rich in tones are not designed to cover hair with a high percentage of white hair. For maximum coverage you should always refer to individual manufacturers' instructions. During the colour consultation make sure you question your client to see if there has been any past incident of colour not taking as well as expected, as this could indicate that the hair is resistant. (See Pre-softening, p. 61)

TIP

Refer to manufacturers' instructions when colouring white hair as there will be a guide on mixing ratios of depth and tone.

PRE-SOFTENING

Pre-softening is a preparation colouring technique: which means that you use it to prepare the hair for a colouring process. In other words, you always use it *before* you apply your target shade. You would use this technique if you conclude from your consultation that your client's hair may be resistant to the permanent colour that you are going to apply to their hair.

Resistant hair has a tightly packed cuticle and a very shiny glassy look; this is common with white hair but can also occur on other types of hair. You would carry out this procedure on colour resistant hair to ensure good coverage and a satisfactory result. If you simply use a straightforward colour technique your colour results may have a faded, wishy-washy appearance which would not be the target shade that you require.

How do I pre-soften?

Apply 20 vol (6%) liquid hydrogen peroxide to the resistant areas using a tinting brush. Place the client under a pre-heated hood dryer for approximately 20 minutes, or you can dry the hydrogen peroxide into the hair with a hand dryer: this added heat will help the hydrogen peroxide to penetrate the cuticle, lifting it enough for the tint (once applied) to penetrate into the cortex. Once you have done this do not rinse out the hydrogen peroxide from the hair, proceed with the tint as normal. Rinse, emulsify and shampoo as normal at the end of the development time.

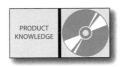

PRODUCT KNOWLEDGE

Pre-softening – products and equipment

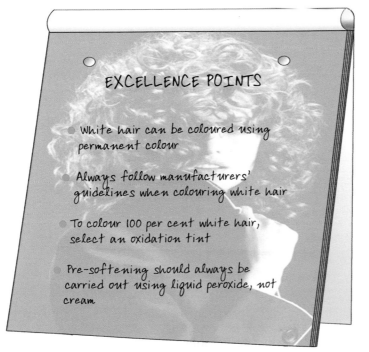

EXCELLENCE POINTS

- White hair can be coloured using permanent colour

- Always follow manufacturers' guidelines when colouring white hair

- To colour 100 per cent white hair, select an oxidation tint

- Pre-softening should always be carried out using liquid peroxide, not cream

TIP ✔

Colour guidance
You must always refer to the individual manufacturers' instructions and the shade chart for guidance. Respect for the recommended development time is essential for a successful and long-lasting colour.

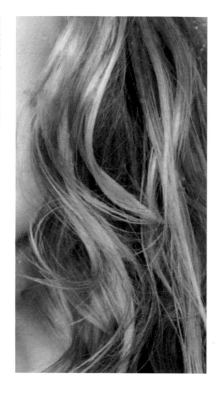

HOW TO ACHIEVE THE CORRECT TARGET SHADE ACCORDING TO THE CLIENT'S NATURAL HAIR COLOUR

There are two natural colour pigments (melanin and pheomelanin) and the natural hair colour we see (black, brown, red or blonde) will depend on the concentration of these pigments within the hair.

When determining the client's natural base we will also need to consider the following:

- What is the percentage of white hair? If the client has a lot of white hair (which can be resistant) you may need to pre-soften the hair (see Pre-softening, p. 61).

- What is the client's required shade?

- How much lighter or darker than their natural colour depth is the shade required?

- How much lift might be expected from the intended artificial colour development?

- Which is the most suitable colouring product to use?

- The strength of the hydrogen peroxide you would use to achieve the result that you require.

- Hair condition and porosity. Remember that some textures of hair can be resistant to colour and porous hair may absorb colour quickly. Take a test cutting if you are unsure about the result. (See Chapter 7)

- Complexion and skin tones. Take into account your client's eye and skin colour and choose a shade together that will complement not distract, e.g. never colour your clients hair too dark or light as this is very ageing.

HEALTH AND SAFETY +

Prepare the client for a colouring/bleaching (pre-lightening) service by gowning the client with a plastic or rubberised tinting gown to protect them from any chemical splashes. The use of towels, plastic shoulder capes and tissues around the neck area will help to ensure your client remains comfortable and protected from any spillages or accidents. If you are using a dark permanent tint or the client has sensitive skin protect the hairline with professional barrier cream.

TIP ✓

Record cards
Remember there is a lot of information needed when colouring and pre-lightening a client's hair, such as the client's name and contact details, date(s) of colour treatments, skin allergy test results, what products and amounts used, the development time and end result. There may be notes on any problems encountered or anything you think would benefit the client on a subsequent colour treatment. Record the details and always complete a record card straight away before you forget any of the details.

Choosing the correct shade

Basic rules are to match up the client's natural root area with the natural depths on the shade chart. Do not look at the ends of the client's hair or at any previously tinted areas as this will not give you the natural depth you are looking for. Once you have established the client's natural depth you need to discuss with them what kind of colour they require. The majority will know what they like by the colour and tone of what they see and will point it out on the shade chart. However, this does not necessarily mean that the particular colour that they have chosen would be suitable for them. This is where your professional skills come into play. You need to work out first whether the shade the client requires is achievable. You do this by taking into account the natural depth, then the artificial colour required by the client, and then work out the difference (if any) of depths. For example if the client's depth is 6 dark blonde and she would like to be 9,3 light golden blonde this is a difference of three levels lighter than her natural colour. Refer to your manufacturer's instructions on the amount of lift that you can get with their products. Usually to achieve three levels of lift you would be using 9% or 30 volume, so in this case the client's choice is achievable. You then need to establish in your professional capacity whether this would suit your client. If you feel the colour is appropriate for them, go ahead, but if you feel that it would look awful and not suit them you must use tact and diplomacy. Make alternative suggestions and compromise constructively, persuading your client as to what would look best on them.

Case study

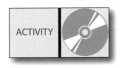

Case study screens

My client wants this colour, what should I do?

- **Case A**
  Natural base 4
  Shade required 4.56
  Answer
  What oxidant would you use?
  Why?

- **Case B**
  Natural base 5
  Shade required 8.34
  Answer
  What oxidant would you use?
  Why?

- **Case C**
  Natural base 6
  Shade required 8
  Answer
  What oxidant would you use?
  Why?

- **Case D**
  Natural base 4
  Shade required 6.64
  Answer
  What oxidant would you use?
  Why?

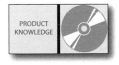

Products

- **Case E**
  Natural base 6
  Shade required 9.03
  Answer
  What oxidant would you use?
  Why?

STEP BY STEP: FULL HEAD TINT APPLICATION

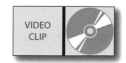

VIDEO CLIP

Steps

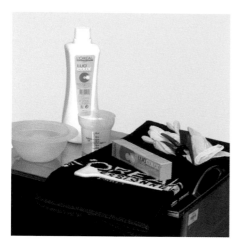

1. Equipment required for application

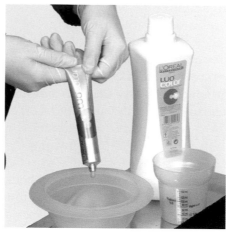

2. Mix products as directed

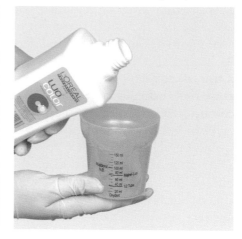

3. Measure required oxidant

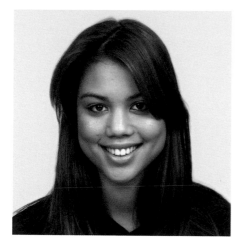

4. Before colour application

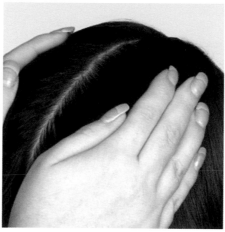

5. Carry out scalp analysis

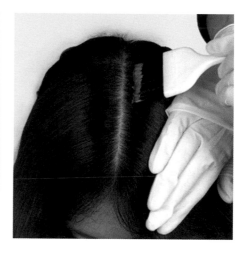

6. Root application

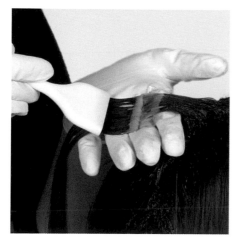

7. Apply to lengths and ends

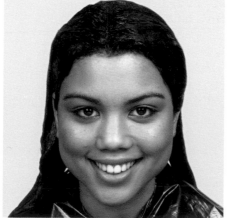

8. Leave for the development time

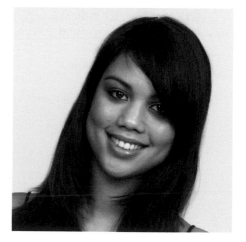

9. Final result

Identifying the hair's artificial colour

When determining the artificial colour of a client's hair we will need to establish the depth and tone of colour remaining in the hair. We will also need to consider if the client requires the same colour that they had last time or a new one.

If the client requires the same colour or wants to add increased tone on the same depth then proceed with the root applicaton and the appropriate colour refreshing technique for the lengths and ends.

If the client wants to reduce the tone or establish a darker colour in the hair then colour correction techniques will need to be applied (see chapter 4). Remember tint will not lighten tint!

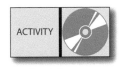

Case study screens

Case study

If you apply this mix, what result will you obtain?

- **Case A**
  Client's natural base: 4
  Oxidant: 20 volumes
  (Hydrogen peroxide strength to be used)
  Permanent tint applied to the client's hair: 6,46

- **Case B**
  Client's natural base: 5
  Oxidant: 20 volumes
  (Hydrogen peroxide strength to be used)
  Permanent tint applied to the client's hair: 7,44

- **Case C**
  Client's natural base: 5
  Oxidant: 20 volumes
  (Hydrogen peroxide strength to be used)
  Permanent tint applied to the client's hair: 7,3

- **Case D**
  Client's natural base: 5
  Oxidant: 30 volumes
  (Hydrogen peroxide strength to be used)
  Permanent tint applied to the client's hair: 8,3

- **Case E**
  Client's natural base: 4
  Oxidant: 20 volumes
  (Hydrogen peroxide strength to be used)
  Permanent tint applied to the client's hair: 7,1

- **Case F**
  Client's natural base: 4
  Oxidant: 30 volumes
  (Hydrogen peroxide strength to be used)
  Permanent tint applied to the client's hair: 8,34

- **Case G**
  Client's natural base: 6
  Oxidant: 20 volumes
  (Hydrogen peroxide strength to be used)
  Permanent tint applied to the client's hair: 8,52

REFRESHING THE LENGTHS AND ENDS WHEN PERMANENTLY COLOURING THE HAIR

Assess the degree of fade on the lengths and ends and select the appropriate refreshing technique for the product you are applying using L'Oréal Professionnel Majirel.

When the colour looks the same

Emulsify the colour:

1 Apply the permanent colour to the regrowth
2 Develop for 35 minutes
3 Add 10–15 mls of warm water to the mixture and emulsify through to the lengths and ends
4 Leave for a further 3–5 minutes.

Tone is missing but the colour is still the same depth

1 Apply permanent colour to the regrowth
2 Develop for 20 minutes
3 Add 10–15 mls warm water to the mixture and immediately apply to lengths and ends
4 Develop for 15–20 minutes.

Colour change same depth – increasing tone

1 Apply permanent colour to the regrowth
2 Add 10–15 mls of warm water to mixture and immediately apply to lengths and ends
3 Develop for 35–40 minutes.

TIP	

Sectioning
Sectioning hair accurately when colouring will ensure methodical completion of the colour, and it will ensure even coverage.

USING ADDED HEAT DURING PERMANENT COLOURING SERVICES

In colouring services heat should only be used if recommended by the manufacturer, *always* refer to instructions. As a rule, added heat will speed up the development time, just as a cold salon will slow down development time.

Heat also radiates from the scalp, making the colouring or bleaching (pre-lightening) product develop quicker at the root area. This will affect your application method and you may have to do a virgin head application which involves applying to the middle lengths and ends first and then the root area to ensure an even result.

TIP
Always be aware of your client's comfort when using added heat.

HEALTH AND SAFETY
Hair condition can become damaged if you use added heat. Do the necessary tests first to assess the hair's condition. (See Chapter 2)

HEALTH AND SAFETY
When working with electrical equipment you are liable under the Electricity at Work regulations so make sure you always label, remove from use and report any faulty electrical equipment which you come across in your workplace.

PERMANENT COLOUR REMOVAL

Once the colour has developed and is ready to be removed, take the client to the backwash. Add a small amount of water then gently massage to loosen the colour using rotary techniques – this is called emulsifying the colour. If massaged thoroughly the tint will be lifted from the scalp and hairline leaving the scalp stain-free.

Rinse until the water runs clear, then shampoo with a pH-balanced shampoo and rinse; a second shampoo should not be necessary.

Apply an anti-oxidant conditioner to close the cuticle, return the hair to its natural pH and to stop the colour fading too quickly.

TIP
pH pH stands for potential hydrogen if you were wondering!

HEALTH AND SAFETY
Always make sure that you do not leave any residue of bleaching (pre-lightening) and colouring products on the hair and scalp at the end of the colouring service as this allows further development of the colour/prelightener, leading to damage to the hair and scalp.

TIP
When removing dark tint from the scalp use a sprinkle of water to begin with and really massage thoroughly. Work on areas such as the front hairline and ears before adding more water. Complete the removal by loosening up from the scalp with the addition of more water, and continue massage and emulsifying before rinsing, shampooing and conditioning.

Why would we use a permanent colour on a client's hair?

- To colour white hair
- To lighten the hair
- To darken the hair
- Add tone to the hair
- To produce a vast range of fashion effects
- To enhance an existing hairstyle
- Change of image

What are the key points to remember when working with permanent colour?

- You cannot lighten tint with tint. Applying a permanent tint on top of a previous permanent colour will not lighten the existing artificial colour
- It can cause an allergic reaction; always do a skin allergy test 48 hours prior to a permanent tint service
- Permanent colour produces a noticeable regrowth, after 4–5 weeks clients will need to make a regular appointment to maintain the colour result
- Permanent colour is not recommended for clients without the commitment to maintain their colour

How long does it last?

After the application of an oxidation colour, a permanent chemical change has occurred within the hair resulting in permanent effects. However, the colour may fade over time due to unsuitable after-care, sensitivity and porosity.

How long should a permanent colouring service take?

When you carry out a colouring service you should be able to work within a 'commercially viable time', these are the industry's guidelines for how long it should take you:

- Mix and apply colour – full head application – 45 minutes maximum
- Mix and apply colour – regrowth – 25 minutes maximum
- Highlights with a cap including preparation and application – 35 minutes maximum
- Woven highlights including preparation and application – 60 minutes maximum

---

TIP

The above timings are the 2003 version of the National Occupational Standards that require individuals to be able to work to a commercially viable time (Habia).

ACTIVITY

Discuss with a group of colleagues why you think it is important to perform all colouring services within commercially acceptable times.

THE EFFECT OF NATURAL AND ARTIFICIAL LIGHT ON PERMANENT COLOUR

Artificial light does not contain the full range of all visible colours that make up natural light. This can affect the apparent colour of the hair. If for example there is no red in the artificial light, the hair cannot reflect red light and may appear colder in colour. In general:

- the light of full daylight shows the true hair colour
- the yellowish light given by some bare electric bulbs adds warmth to hair colour, but neutralises blue or ash colour effects
- the bluish light produced by some fluorescent tubes tends to neutralise the warmth of red hair colours.

Facts about natural light

- The visible spectrum comprises all of the colours that can be seen by the human eye
- When all colours are reflected from a surface it looks white
- When all colours are absorbed by a surface it looks black
- When one colour is reflected from a surface and the rest are absorbed, it is the colour that is reflected that we see, e.g. a ripe tomato absorbs all light except red, which it reflects.
- Due to the hair's ability to reflect part of the visible spectrum, the true hair colour can only be seen in natural daylight.

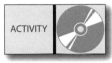

The effect of natural and artificial light

Achieving the desired colouring effect, which is to the satisfaction of your client.
Giving your client suitable advice on the maintenance of their permanent colour

Confirming the desired effect with your client prior to the application of colour

Sectioning the hair cleanly and evenly, when necessary, to assist the accurate application of colouring and lightening products

Identifying any problems during the colouring process and resolving them within the limits of your own authority to do so. Referring problems which cannot be resolved to the relevant person promptly

Permanently change hair colour by

Applying colouring and lightening products accurately, taking into account relevant factors influencing the service

Removing colouring materials from hair to minimise discomfort to your client.
Leaving the hair and scalp free of colouring products after the desired effect is achieved

Using colour application techniques suitable for achieving the desired look. Applying colour in a way that minimises the risk of the product being spread to your client's skin, clothes and surrounding areas

Confirming the required colour result has been achieved by taking strand tests at suitable times throughout the process. Removing products that have been developed from the hair, avoiding disturbance to areas still processing

Using colouring and lightening products, and accurately timing the development of the colour following the manufacturer's instructions

EXCELLENCE POINTS

- The higher the strength of oxidant, the more lift can be obtained

- Permanent tint lightens and colours at the same time

- Each depth of colour corresponds to an undercoat

- Always carry out a skin allergy test 48 hours before providing a permanent colour service

BLEACHING (PRE-LIGHTENING) HAIR

How do bleaches (pre-lighteners) work?

All bleaching products (pre-lighteners) are alkaline and contain ammonia. The alkali in bleach (pre-lightener) has two actions:

- It mixes with the hydrogen peroxide and releases the oxygen, which will oxidise the melanin into oxy-melanin and pheomelanin into colourless oxy-pheomelanin, lightening the base (depth) colour.
- It swells the hair and opens up the cuticle so that the bleach (pre-lightener) can penetrate into the cortex.

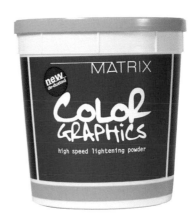

What effect do lightening products have on the hair structure?

- A **lightening product** contains ammonia and persalts. On contact with an oxidant, it is going to release oxygen which will oxidise the natural pigments and produce a level of lightening/undercoat on the hair.
- L'Oréal Professionnel cream oxidants come in three concentrations: **20, 30** and **40 volumes**. This means that they can release 20, 30 or 40 times their oxygen volume. It is the volume of released oxygen which determines the lightening strength. An oxidant can also be characterised in terms of percentage: 6%, 9% or 12%. In other words, it contains 6%, 9% or 12% of oxygen.
- According to its volume/percentage, the oxygen released gradually lightens the granular pigments, followed by that of the diffused pigments.
- The more the oxidant and the lightening product release oxygen, the paler the level of lightening/undercoat will be.

HEALTH AND SAFETY

Potential risks when using powder bleach (pre-lightener)
Do not inhale as the associated dangers are:

- Damage to mucal tissues of mouth and nose
- Respiratory tract damage
- Damage to the lungs.

How long does it last?

- Using a bleaching (pre-lightening) product on a client's hair is a chemical process that will create a permanent change within the hair structure until it grows out or is cut off.

Bleach (pre-lightener) is used to lighten hair when other products such as high-lift tints cannot give you the light blonde you require. It is practically impossible to obtain lighter than pale yellow except when you use strong bleaching (pre-lightening) products. These are able to produce a greater amount of oxygen, which oxides the diffuse (pheomelanin) pigment.

BLEACHING (PRE-LIGHTENING) PRODUCTS

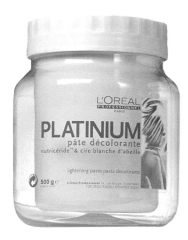

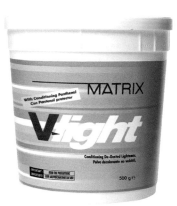

A selection of bleach (pre-lightening) products

Emulsion bleach

Emulsion bleach is made up of three separate components:

- Oil or gel bleach
- Boosters or activators
- Hydrogen peroxide.

Always read the manufacturer's instructions before using this product to determine the recommended strength of hydrogen peroxide and the number of boosters/activators you must use.

Make sure that you mix it in the order specified or it will be ineffective and curdle.

Emulsion bleaches are especially formulated to be kind to the scalp so these products are particularly good for full head and regrowth bleach (pre-lightener) clients.

Development of bleach (pre-lightener) is by observation, which means that you must monitor the different stages of lightening by watching and conducting strand tests at regular intervals.

> **TIP**
>
> **Bleach strand test**
> - When performing the strand test carefully remove all the bleach with a dry piece of cotton wool.
> - Many bleach products have a blue colour effect; this can make the hair appear lighter than it actually is as blue neutralises yellow.
> - Once you have a piece of clean hair it will give you an accurate 'reading' of the level of the lift achieved.

Powder bleach (pre-lightening) products

Powder bleach (pre-lightening) products are mixed with hydrogen peroxide (20 vol [6%] or 30 vol [9%]). The strength that you choose will depend on the amount of lift that you require. Powder bleaches (prc-lighteners) can be fast-developing products, you will need to be careful to monitor development at all times to ensure that it is not exceeding the required lift, as this could result in damage to the hair or scalp.

Powder bleaches (pre-lighteners) are mixed to a smooth paste, but always read the manufacturer's instructions as the strength of hydrogen-peroxide will vary with different products and whether you are using liquid or cream peroxide.

Some powder bleaches (pre-lighteners) are more suited for highlights (cap and foil) and fashion effects. Some can damage the scalp and are not as suitable for a full head bleach (pre-lightener); however, other powder bleaches can be used on the scalp, so always check the manufacturer's instructions.

CHOOSING THE CORRECT BLEACHING (PRE-LIGHTENING) PRODUCT FOR YOUR CLIENT

For each level of colour, there is a corresponding level of lightening (undercoat) (See page 50). These levels of lightening go from red, colour level 1, to very pale yellow, colour level 10. Depending on the amount of lightening required there are several products and technologies.

Removal of a bleach (pre-lightener)

When you are removing a full head bleach (pre-lightener) be very careful with the temperature of the water as the client's scalp may be sensitive. Emulsion bleach is designed to be gentle on the scalp but it may still be delicate.

Run cool water through the hair (always protecting the client's eyes) until you have rinsed most of the bleach (pre-lightener) away, do not massage the scalp at this stage. Gently rinse and shampoo the hair.

HEALTH AND SAFETY

Chemically treated hair

Potential dangers to the hair structure of using bleach (pre-lightening) and colouring products on chemically treated hair include increased damage to the cuticle and cortex: the cuticle could become more porous making the hair feel dry and lifeless, or the cortex could lose elasticity causing the hair to break and split and lead to disintegration. It could also lead to an uneven and unsatisfactory colour result, a possible incompatibility of products and reaching the result sooner than expected. When you bleach (pre-lighten) hair, it lightens in different stages. You should never lighten a client's hair beyond a very pale yellow undercoat: beyond this, the hair fibre could be attacked which can cause severe breakage of the hair. Refer to your Levels of lightening chart on p. 50.

EXCELLENCE POINTS

- Never over-lighten as this will affect the hair fibre

- Always check the lightening process frequently

- Always follow the manufacturer's instructions carefully

- Ensure that protective garments are worn by you and your client

STEP BY STEP: FULL HEAD BLEACH (PRE-LIGHTENER) APPLICATION

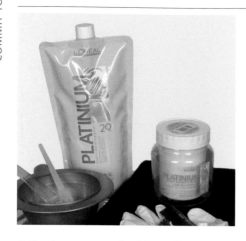

1. Equipment required for colour application

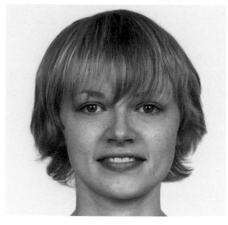

2. Before colour application

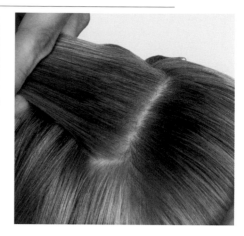

3. Analyse the hair and scalp

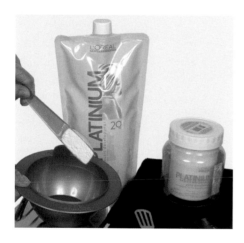

4. Mix product according to the manufacturer's instructions

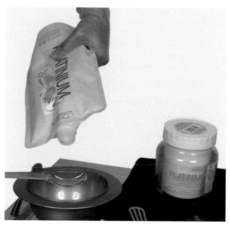

5. Measure the required oxidant

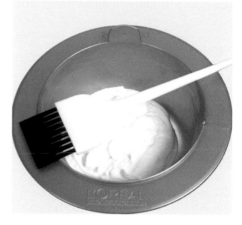

6. Clean tools will ensure ease of application

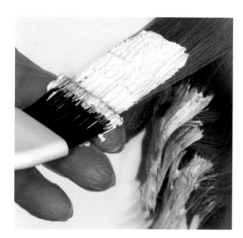

7. Make the application to the lengths and ends of the hair, starting at the nape area and working upwards towards the crown

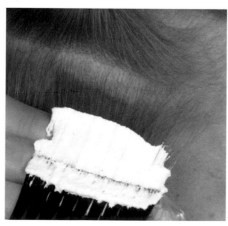

8. Continue the application to the lengths and ends, when complete, begin the root application

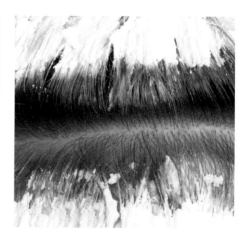

9. Make application to the roots, overlapping to the lengths and ends to refresh product

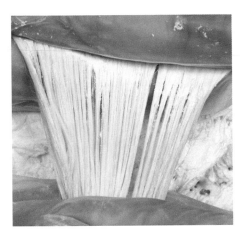

10. Monitor constantly until degree of lift has been achieved. Always develop in accordance with the manufacturer's instructions

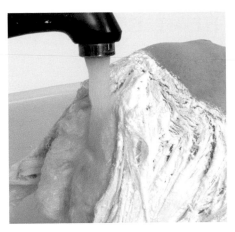

11. Rinse with tepid water and shampoo gently

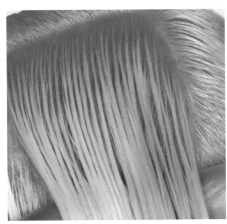

12. Analyse the bleaching (pre-lightening) result in order to select the correct tonal shade

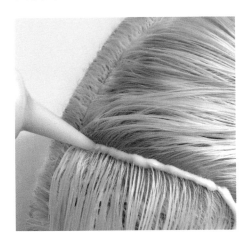

13. Apply toner quickly and evenly throughout the hair

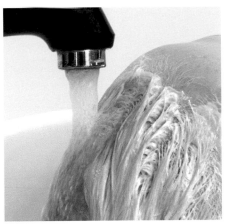

14. Rinse, emulsify and shampoo gently

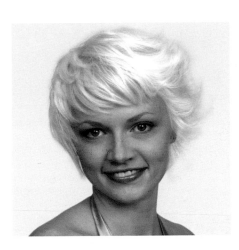

15. Final colour result

VIDEO CLIP

Steps

PRODUCT KNOWLEDGE

Product

TIP ✓

When lengths and ends application is complete, ensure that you have achieved half of the required level of lift before commencing a root application.

TIP ✓

All factors relating to the client's hair and scalp must be taken into consideration before any bleaching (pre-lightening) application.

STEP BY STEP: CAP HIGHLIGHTS

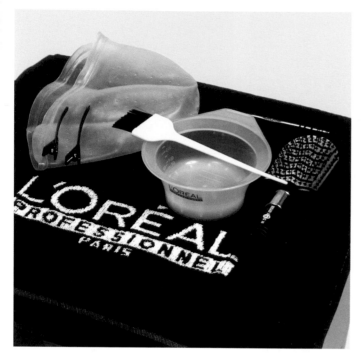

1. Equipment required for cap highlights

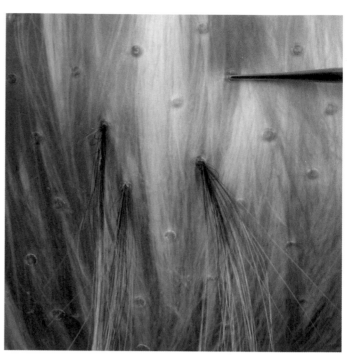

2. Identify the highlight area

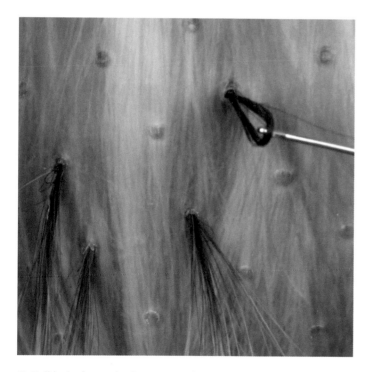

3. Pull hair through the cap as shown

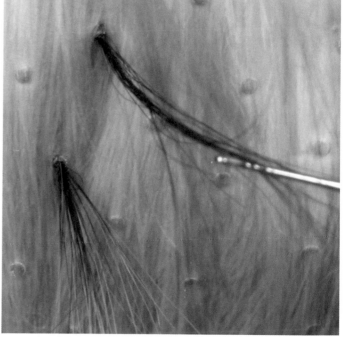

4. Continue until sufficient highlights have been pulled through the cap

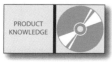

Steps

STEP BY STEP: FULL HEAD HIGHLIGHTS APPLICATION

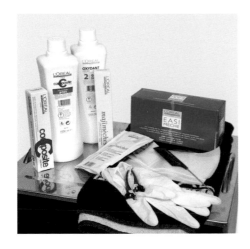

1. Equipment required for colour application

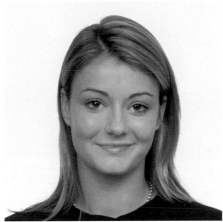

2. Before colour application

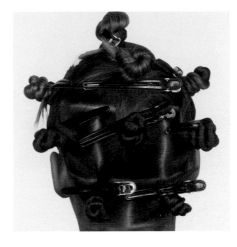

3. Prepare the hair by sectioning

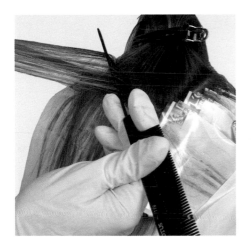

4. Take a fine section of hair

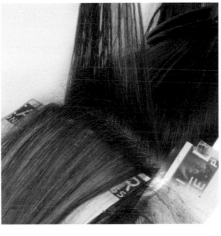

5. Weave close to the scalp

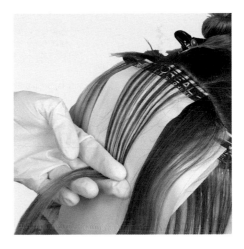

6. Place meche or foil underneath woven section

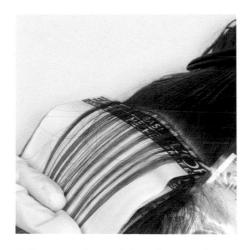

7. Keep meche or foil as close to the root as possible

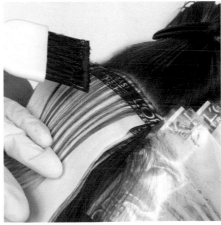

8. Paint product on hair

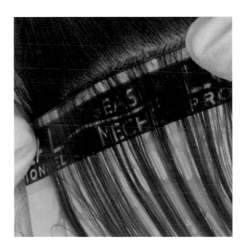

9. Close meche or foil by sealing at corners

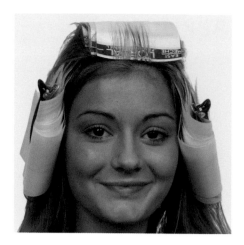

10. Leave for full development time

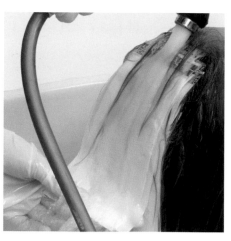

11. Rinse meches or foils to remove, emulsify and shampoo as normal

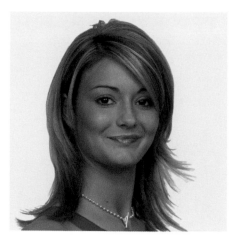

12. Final result

PRODUCT KNOWLEDGE

Products

VIDEO CLIP

Steps

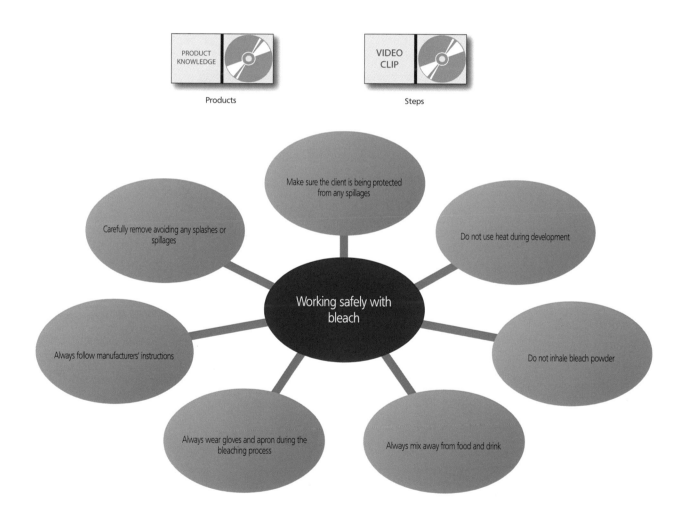

Make sure the client is being protected from any spillages

Carefully remove avoiding any splashes or spillages

Do not use heat during development

Always follow manufacturers' instructions

Working safely with bleach

Do not inhale bleach powder

Always wear gloves and apron during the bleaching process

Always mix away from food and drink

HEALTH AND SAFETY ✚

Mixing powder bleach (pre-lighteners)
When mixing powder pre-lighteners it is very important to ensure that there are no lumps as these could create 'hot spots' on the hair during development, causing hair breakage.

TIP

Always apply a pH-balanced conditioner to the hair as this will close the cuticle, return the hair to its natural pH state and help prevent colour fade.

ACTIVITY

Take nine cuttings of hair (save hair from the salon floor when a client has had a lot of hair cut off) mix up some powder bleach (pre-lightener) with 9% or 30 volume and apply to all nine cuttings of hair using nine pieces of foil to rest the hair on. After five minutes remove the bleach from one of the cuttings, after 10 minutes remove the bleach from the second piece of hair and every five minutes after that until the last piece of hair has had the bleach on for 40 minutes. Stick and label the different cuttings of hair from the darkest to the lightest. This will give you a good idea of all the different stages of bleaching.

TIP

When you are removing foil highlights where some of the hair is still developing, be very careful not to disturb the hair that is still processing as some of the product contained in the packets could seep and leak onto the rest of the hair causing an uneven 'tiger stripe' effect.

TIP

When you are getting all your tools and equipment ready for your colouring client it is essential to position them so they are easy for you to reach: this will make your job a lot easier and promotes an efficient service. This in turn will instill confidence in your client, promoting a trusting relationship. Keeping your work area clean and tidy will also promote a professional relationship, minimise the risk of cross-infection and reduce hazards.

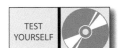

Common problems and solutions

Troubleshooting: common colouring problems and solutions

Colouring problem	Cause	Action
Over-processing with permanent colour or bleach (pre-lightener)	Product left on too long Hydrogen peroxide too strong	Use penetrating conditioner or restructuring treatments
Under-processing with colour permanent or bleach (pre-lightener)	Product not left on long enough Not enough product applied Hydrogen peroxide too weak	If hair condition allows it reapply bleach (pre-lightener) or colour
Skin staining	Too much product applied Poor application Failure to protect the skin Ineffective removal	Clean using stain remover
Deterioration of hair condition	Colouring product too strong Over-processing Hydrogen peroxide too strong	Use penetrating conditioning treatments

Troubleshooting: common colouring problems and solutions (continued)

Colouring problem	Cause	Action
Uneven result	Uneven application	Re-application of product (spot colour)
	Uneven porosity	Use pre-treatments prior to next colour or bleach
	Incorrect product used	(pre-lightener) application to help to even out porosity
	Incorrect use of heat	
	Incorrect mixing	
Product seepage	Too much product applied	Spot colour/spot weave affected areas
	Packets not secured correctly	
Scalp irritation	Allergy or sensitivity to product	Remove product immediately and rinse with cool water
	Product too strong	Seek medical advice
Hair breakage	Over processing	Remove immediately
	Poor porosity	Use restructurant
		Use penetrating conditioner

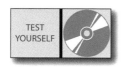

TEST YOURSELF

Testing and essential knowledge

Assessment of knowledge and understanding

Test yourself on the content of this chapter by answering these questions. This will help you to prepare for your Essential knowledge/Written test.

1 How would you gown and protect your client before a permanent colouring service? List three available protective clothing materials that you would use on your client and state why it is important to use this equipment before a colouring service.

2 What tests would it be necessary to carry out on your client's hair before carrying out a permanent colouring service?

3 List the details you would need to complete a record card for your colouring client, and state when is the ideal time to complete it.

4 How long should it take you to carry out the following services:

(a) Mix and apply a full head colour

(b) Mix and apply a regrowth colour

(c) Highlights using a cap including preparation

(d) Woven highlights including preparation?

5 How would you correctly dispose of left over colour or bleach (pre-lightener)?

6 For each of the following colouring and lightening problems you need one possible cause, one way of resolving the problem, how you would resolve the problem within your own limits of authority and who would you report the problem to if you cannot resolve it. Copy the table below and add your answers.

Problem	Cause	Resolving problem	Authority	Person to report to
Over-processing with colour or bleach				
Under-processing with colour or bleach				
Skin staining				
Deterioration of hair condition				
Uneven result				
Product seepage				

7 What are your responsibilities under the current Electricity at Work Act?

8 How can the position of your client affect the desired outcome of the service and lead to fatigue and injury?

9 Describe seven methods of working safely and hygienically when colouring and bleaching (pre-lightening) hair.

10 State three reasons why it is important to restore freshly coloured hair to its natural pH?

11 State two reasons why it is important to section the hair accurately when applying colour.

12 Draw and describe two line diagrams demonstrating how permanent colour and bleach affects the hair structure. How long does each of these types of colour last?

13 Work out the ratio of water that you would need to achieve the different strengths of hydrogen peroxide by completing the table below.

	Dilute to	Answer
12%	6%	
18%	9%	
9%	6%	

14 State two reasons why it is important to remove all traces of colouring and bleaching (pre-lightening) products from the hair at the end of each colouring service.

15 Think of two reasons why it is important to avoid disturbing areas that are still processing when removing products from developed areas.

16 Name the different bleaching (pre-lightening) products available and state the best use for each.

17 Describe the potential damaging effects to the cuticle and cortex of the hair when using bleaching (pre-lightening) and colouring products on chemically treated hair.

18 Describe how granular pigment (melanin) creates natural hair colour.

19 How does (a) natural light and (b) artificial light affect the appearance of colour?

20 How does natural colour affect the colouring process?

21 How do different strengths of hydrogen peroxide affect the hair colouring and bleaching (pre-lightening) process?

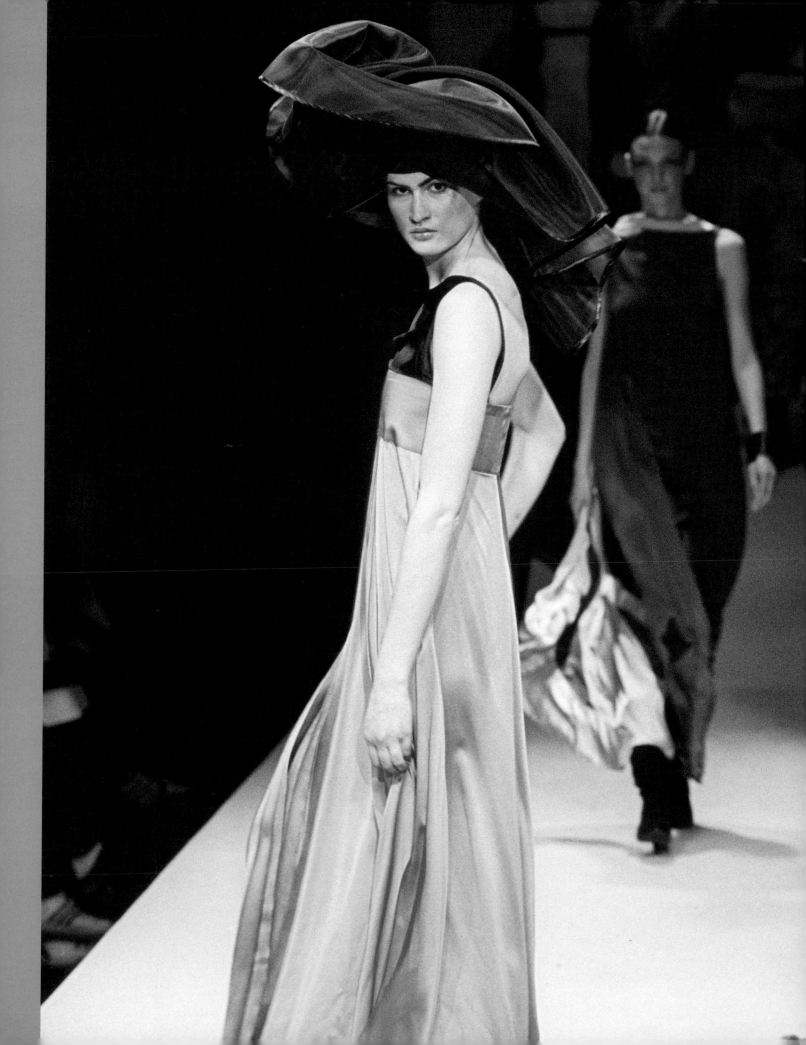

Colour change

Everyone has a dream, and if you're reading this, you're lucky enough to be on your way to making it reality. It may be your dream to be a celebrity stylist flying between Milan and New York, to build your own business, or to work in your local salon. Whatever your direction, it's your dream and your motivation that will get you there.

Whichever path you choose, an 'it'll do' attitude may be easy, but it's not very challenging. It's one of the quickest routes to boredom. You may even get a lot of clients – once. You're going into an industry that's buzzing with new ideas, innovative techniques and products. To excel is to keep up to speed with all that's going on, to know your product, to perfect your skill. To excel is to want to be the very best you can.

'Once clients have experienced the joy of how hair colour can change their look, lift their appearance, make them look younger, complement their hair cut, they'll be hooked.' For Jo Hansford, one of the UK's top colourists, colour is the 'best high in the world'. That must be one of the clearest definitions of success, to make someone feel that good about themselves. To succeed is to follow a career that you're passionate about, that challenges you to your best every day.

chapter 4

COLOUR CHANGE

Learning objectives

In this chapter, you will learn how to assess your client's hair and perform 'expert eyes' analysis to identify the corrective treatment required for you to provide them with their dream colour. In *colour change*, we will consider:

- **The power of change**

- **The principles of colour correction**

- **How to offer an expert service**

- **Communication techniques**

- **Expert eyes detailed analysis**

- **The colour wheel in colour correction**

- **The principles of relative tones**

- **Contraindications and their effect on colour correction**

- **Colour reduction**

- **Reduction and oxidation**

- **Pre-softening colour resistant hair**

- **Colour-in or pre-pigmentation**

- **Colouring, bleaching and lightening problems and remedial actions**

H28 Provide colour correction services

THE POWER OF CHANGE

Colour change is your passport to knowing how to propose and to put into practice, in the salon, with full confidence, all aspects of colour correction/change. Simply change the tone, darken or lighten, master special effects and many accessible creative and commercial techniques so that 'colour change' becomes an everyday salon service, not only creative but profitable.

Remember change is the reason we are in the hairdressing industry, and changing and personalising a client's look can be as easy as changing any other fashion accessory.

How does it feel when you change a client's colour? The client feels great, your colleagues comment on how good your work is. You enjoy what you do more.

Changing a client's colour is exciting and motivating. It is up to us to offer a change to the client.

THE PRINCIPLES OF COLOUR CHANGE/CORRECTION

Before we move on to colour correction we need to know what it is and why we do it. Colour correction consists of three main principles:

1   Hair that needs to be lightened if it is too dark
2   Hair that needs to be darkened if it is too light
3   Changing the unwanted existing artificial colour tone to suit the client.

This does not necessarily mean that colour correction has to be a long drawn-out affair: it could turn out to be a quick process, so assessing the client's hair correctly is very important.

HOW TO OFFER AN EXPERT SERVICE

Offer an expert service by:

- Assessing a client's hair prior to colour correction
- Communication.

Assessing a client's hair prior to colour correction

It is very important when dealing with a colour correction service that you assess the hair correctly before proceeding. It is often the case that a client needing a remedial colouring service will not be entirely truthful or knowledgeable when questioned as to what has happened to their hair. This may be due to embarrassment, or just the urgency to get their hair back to a satisfactory colour result.

Remember that colour change can seem scary but do not panic – you have the knowledge to fix it!

Assessing a client's hair prior to colour correction

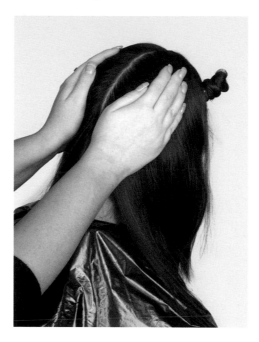 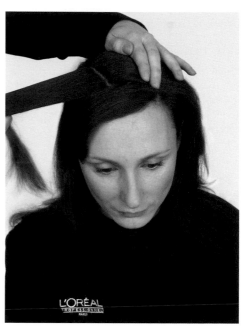

Communication techniques

Communication is a natural thing that we do every day. When we talk to friends and family, we feel confident and tend to communicate well. However, when we talk with clients who are new to the salon there can be an uncertainty in the communication because we do not know them very well. You can talk at cross-purposes and not get to the bottom of what your client requires: this will lead to dissatisfaction with the service and the loss of a client.

Let us look a little more deeply at what we should and should not say to encourage a client to talk to us, and how to build a trusting relationship between you and your client. When we communicate with our clients there is a sequence that we need to go through in order to gain the right information and present a professional service.

There is a beginning, middle and end to this process.

Beginning

Introduce yourself to your client, for example:

'Hello my name is …….. I am going to do your hair today! Can I begin by asking a few questions?'

Middle

Use open, confirmation and closed questions.

End

The conclusion: you listen and reiterate back to your client. Listen to what your client says and then reformulate the answer for her. 'So if I understand you correctly you said ... and ... Therefore I will...'

Here are some initial positive questions to ask your client

- *How did you like your last colour?*
  This gives you a good idea of her satisfaction

- *Do you want to keep the same colour?*
  This will lead the client to give you more information

- *What type of shades don't you like?*
  This will help to eliminate what she dislikes

- *So you like warm shades?*
  This will confirm what the client wishes

- *So you would prefer a slightly lighter shade?*
  This will help to confirm what the client desires

- *What do you think about this shade?*
  This will indicate if you are on the right track

- *Do you want to darken it a little?*
  This will indicate if you are on the right track

- *What do you think about a few lighter highlights?*
  This will open the door to a new proposal

- *Would you like a change?*
  This will open the door to a new proposal

- *So you prefer subtle effects?*
  Confirms that you are listening to her

- *What don't you like about this shade?*
  This will eliminate what she does not like

- *What colours do you like wearing?*
  This will help to confirm your client's image

- *How do you feel about your hair today?*
  This opens the door to dialogue

- *So if I understand correctly....?*
  This confirms the client's desires

Questions that are to be avoided

- *Who did this colour for you?*
  Criticism of her choice of colourist or your competitors

- *Do you want the same colour?*
  Leaves her little choice, you do not have time for her

- *Shall I do the same as usual?*
  She might not dare to say that she no longer likes what you do

- *Do you want the same thing as me?*
  Difficult to tell you she does not like your colour

- *Do you know what you had the last time?*
  You should be telling the client that, not the other way around – you're the professional!

- *What mixture did you have the last time?*
  This is unprofessional. You must keep accurate and up-to-date client records

- *What would you like me to do for you?*
  Closes the door on a new proposal

- *Do you know what you want?*
  Closes the door on a new proposal

- *Do you trust me?*
  It is asking your client to take a leap of faith that they might not be ready to take

- *Do you do your own colour?*
  This could be taken as an insult

- *Do you want classic highlights?*
  No one sees himself or herself as classic

- *How about a few streaks?*
  This provides the client with no indication of the finished result

- *Leave it to me?*
  It is asking your client to take risks

When to use open, confirmation and closed questions

Now that you know about the types of questions that you can ask the client, let's look at how to put it all together.

Open questions	Confirmation questions	Closed questions
If you need information from your client use questions that begin with Who, How, What, Where, Would and When. These will lead to more information as opposed to a 'Yes' 'No' answer	Ask this type of question when you need verification from your client	Use this type of question when you need a definite 'Yes' or 'No' from your client
1 How did you like your last colour? This gives you a good idea of her satisfaction	1 What type of shades don't you like? This will help to eliminate what she does not like	1 Do you want to keep the same colour? This will lead to more information
2 What do you think about this shade? This will indicate if you are on the right track	2 So you prefer subtle effects? Confirms that you are listening to her	2 So you like warm shades? This will confirm what the client wishes
3 What do you think about a few lighter highlights? This will open the door to a new proposal	3 What don't you like about this shade? This will eliminate what she does not like	3 So you would prefer a slightly lighter shade? This will confirm what the client wishes
4 Would you like a change? This will open the door to a new proposal	4 So if I understand correctly....? This confirms the client's desires	4 Do you want to darken it a little? This will indicate if you are on the right track

Questioning

Always question the client thoroughly to find out:

- What previous hairdressing treatments have they had on their hair?
- Have they any history of allergic reaction to chemical treatments?
- Are they currently taking any medication, or just recently finished?
- Have they received any medical advice that would contraindicate a colouring service?
- How would they like the finished result to look (using a shade chart)?
- Have they used any home colouring products?

Testing the hair

You should always test the hair before attempting any colour correction to assess the general condition of the hair and scalp. To learn or recap on how to carry out hair sensitivity testing, refer to Chapter 1.

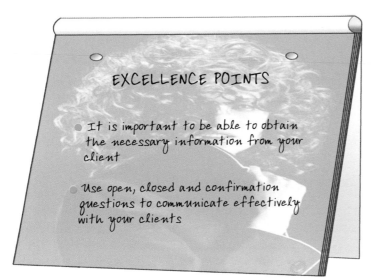

EXCELLENCE POINTS

- It is important to be able to obtain the necessary information from your client

- Use open, closed and confirmation questions to communicate effectively with your clients

EXPERT EYES – DETAILED ANALYSIS

Using your expert eyes, you will need to assess:

- What is the present situation regarding your client's natural and artificial colour?

- What is the natural base of your client's hair?
  Use your shade chart to help to confirm this. When you become experienced with colour, you will be able to work out the natural depth/base just by looking at the natural root area of the hair.

- What is the length of the regrowth?
  For example, L'Oréal Professionnel colour is designed to work best with the natural scalp temperature of 37 degrees. When the regrowth is over 1 cm colour does not benefit from the natural heat of the scalp. Therefore, the colour may not develop to the correct level and tone. In this situation, we may need to pre-soften the additional regrowth area – see Chapter 3.

- What percentage of the hair is white?

- What is the colour history of your client's hair?
  What colours do you see in their hair? What depth and tone? Have they any hidden blonde highlights, for example? Ask detailed questions to help you to find out what colours have been applied to your client's hair.

- What artificial colour is visible on the lengths and ends?
  Again, use your shade chart and take into account the amount of fade that may have occurred since the last colour application.

- What is the length of your client's hair?
  If your client has below-shoulder-length hair, you must consider any colour applications made over the last three years.

HEALTH AND SAFETY

Skin allergy tests
It is very important to ensure that you are carrying out skin allergy tests on all permanent colour clients 48 hours, or as per the manufacturer's instructions, prior to colour service being carried out. This will identify any allergic reaction, helping you to uphold your professional responsibilities to health and safety and other legislation, thus maintaining the professional image of the salon.

- How long since the last application? When did your client last apply a colour to their hair?
- Hair sensitivity – How porous and damaged is the hair due to chemical, heat and mechanical abuse?
- What is the client's desired shade or their 'dream' colour? What colours do they want to see in their hair?

You can now decide what technique you will use to achieve this.

Course of action following consultation

To help you to establish the correct colour service to be carried out, always record your findings and the client's responses for your future records: this also provides you with documented evidence of the client's initial consultation for future colour services. Use record cards or detailed analysis (see examples below) to help you store your client's information.

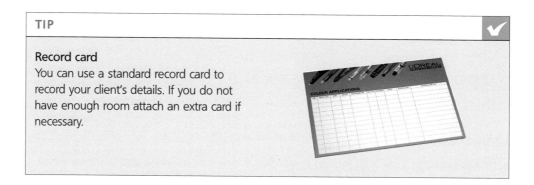

TIP ✔

Record card
You can use a standard record card to record your client's details. If you do not have enough room attach an extra card if necessary.

Remember to be honest with yourself and your client, even if the conclusion of the consultation is not what the client wants to hear. It is far better to have a client happy in the long term than short-term fixes that could damage the hair, further creating more problems. Always give your client the best advice you can so you can agree a plan of action to restore your clients colour.

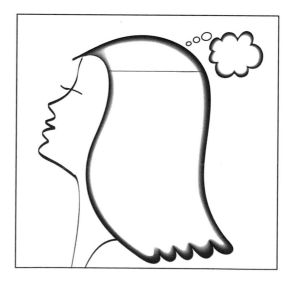

Natural Base	
% of White	
Length of regrowth	
Level on lengths / ends	L / E
Reflect on lengths /ends	L / E
Desired shade	
Compatibility of reflects	
Ideal Undercoat	

THE COLOUR WHEEL IN COLOUR CORRECTION

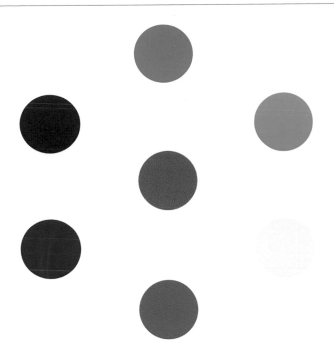

The colour wheel

Using a shade chart identifies the existing artificial depth and tone of your client's hair, using the colour wheel will identify the best colour to neutralise unwanted tones.

The colour wheel consists of primary and secondary colours:

- Primary colours are blue, red and yellow
- Secondary colours are green, purple and orange.

For more information about the colour wheel, see Chapter 3.

The colour wheel is used during colour correction. Opposite colours on the wheel will neutralise unwanted tones, so for example:

If a client's highlights are too brassy and orange, by using a blue ash tonal shade the excess warmth will be neutralised.

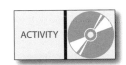

The colour wheel

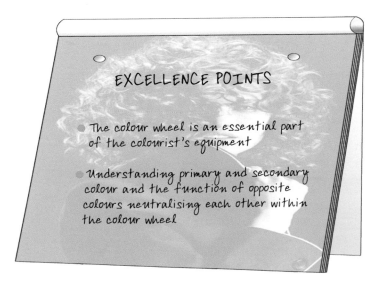

EXCELLENCE POINTS

- The colour wheel is an essential part of the colourist's equipment

- Understanding primary and secondary colour and the function of opposite colours neutralising each other within the colour wheel

THE PRINCIPLE OF RELATIVE TONES

When you are changing the tone of your client's hair, you must consider whether the tone that you will be adding to the hair will be compatible with the existing artificial tone that is already present in the hair.

First, we need to recap the tones used for colouring. For example, below is L'Oréal Professionnel's tonal numbering system.

blue ash	mauve ash (iridescent)	gold	copper	mahogany	red	metallic
,1	,2	,3	,4	,5	,6	,7

Please refer to Chapter 3 for more information on tones.

In order to decide what tones are compatible, you just need to think about colour and imagine what happens when you mix colours together, then you have your answer to compatible or not. In other words, if I put this gold on my client's brown hair will it come out gold?

For example:

Compatible result

Existing colour	Orange
Required shade	Red
Result	Red

Incompatible result

Existing colour	Gold
Required shade	Green
Result	Lime green

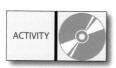

ACTIVITY

Use the Daisy Wheel to check compatibility

Case study

The client's existing tone is ,3 gold
The client wishes to become a ,4 copper
Will the addition of copper over gold produce a true copper tone?
Answer: Yes

Therefore, these tones are compatible.

The client's existing tone is ,1 blue (ash)
The client wishes to become a ,3 gold
Will the addition of ,3 gold over the ,1 blue (ash) produce a true gold tone?
Answer: No

Therefore, these tones are not compatible.

ACTIVITY

Is there compatibility?

Case	Existing Reflect		Desired Reflect		Yes	No	Not Sure
1	Copper	.4	Red	.6			
2	Metallic	.7	Gold	.3			
3	Copper	.4	Mahogany	.5			
4	Ash	.1	Gold	.3			
5	Iridescent	.2	Red	.6			
6	Red	.6	Mahogany	.5			
7	Copper	.4	Gold	.3			
8	Red	.6	Iridescent	.2			
9	Ash	.1	Red	.6			
10	Mahogany	.5	Gold	.3			
11	Iridescent	.2	Copper	.4			
12	Ash	.1	Mahogany	.5			
13	Gold	.3	Mahogany	.5			
14	Copper	.4	Ash	.1			
15	Mahogany	.5	Red	.6			
16	Red	.6	Gold	.3			

But what about double tones?

For example:

.46 – Copper red   .51 – Mahogany ash
.34 – Gold copper   .35 – Golden mahogany

- These colours are a delicate combination of different tones, which give fashion shades.
- Even with a combination of tones the principle of compatibility does not change.
- If any one of the four tones is incompatible, the desired colour will not be achieved and the end result will be incorrect.

Let us see if you can work out if these double tones are compatible or incompatible.

ACTIVITY

Double Reflects

Existing Shade	Desired Shade	Compatible	Incompatible	Not Sure
8.31	8.34			
7.1	7.43			
6.34	6.46			
5.12	5.52			
8.13	8.42			
7.44	7.31			
5.4	5.64			

Important note: If ash tones are present in the hair, they will need to be removed before re-colouring.

Now we can answer the question of compatibility of tones on the detailed analysis we can select what would be the most suitable colour change/correction technique to use.

Which technique do we use when the tones are compatible?

Compatibility of tones ⟶ Yes ⟶ Colour-in ⟶ Chosen technique = Take Through Immediately

What does this mean?

If the existing artificial tone is compatible with the new artificial tone that you are going to apply to your client's hair then you can use the technique Take Through Immediately.

How do I Take Through Immediately?

- Apply the desired shade to the roots
- Add 15 mls of warm water to the remaining mixture
- Take through immediately to the lengths and ends
- Develop for 35 minutes
- Remember: if 30 volume oxidant has been used on the roots, you must mix fresh product with 20 volume for the lengths and ends.

Which technique would we use if the tones are not compatible?

Compatibility of tones ⟶ No ⟶ Colour-out ⟶ Chosen technique = Cleanse

If your client has chosen a new colour which is incompatible with her existing tone the old tone will need to be removed. This technique is called 'cleanse'. To do this you will need to use a product designed to remove permanent colour pigment to remove any unwanted tone or build up of colour.

How do I cleanse?

To remove tone using L'Oréal Professionnel Efassor:

- In a non-metallic bowl, mix 1 packet of Efassor with 60mls of hot water
- Place this bowl in another bowl of hot water
- Apply quickly with a sponge to the lengths and ends at the backwash
- Massage well until the tone has been removed (up to 20 minutes)
- Rinse and shampoo
- Lightly dry
- Apply the target shade to the root area
- Add 15mls of warm water to the remaining mixture
- Take through immediately to the lengths and ends
- Develop for 35 minutes.

STEP BY STEP: GENTLE CLEANSE

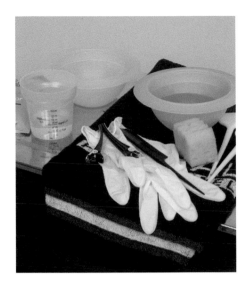

1. Equipment required for a gentle cleanse

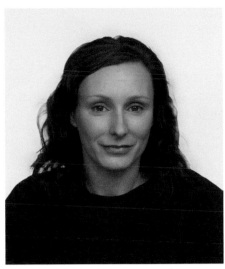

2. Before colour reduction

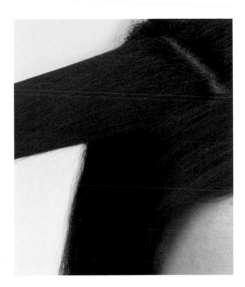

3. Analyse the hair to determine the colour reduction required

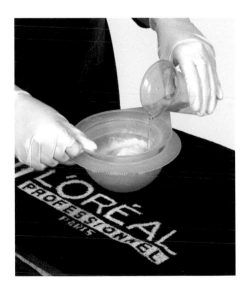

4. Mix product as directed

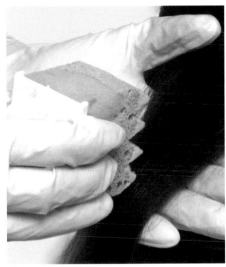

5. Using a sponge, apply to lengths and ends

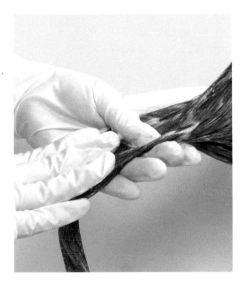

6. Gently massage until level of reduction is achieved

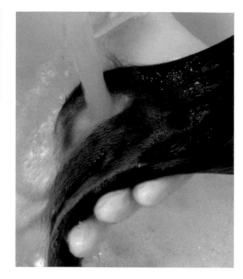

7. Rinse and shampoo

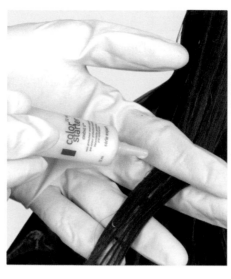

8. Apply porosity leveller to sensitised areas if necessary

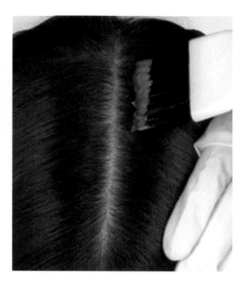

9. Apply chosen shade to the root area

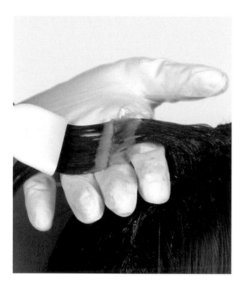

10. Apply to lengths and ends

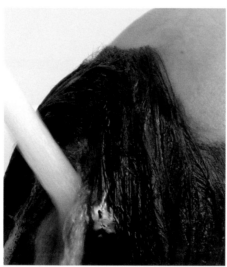

11. Emulsify, rinse and shampoo

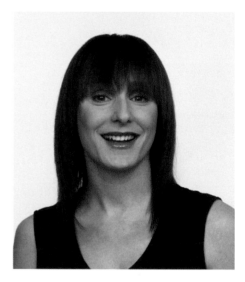

12. Final result

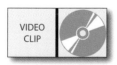

Steps

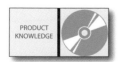

Product

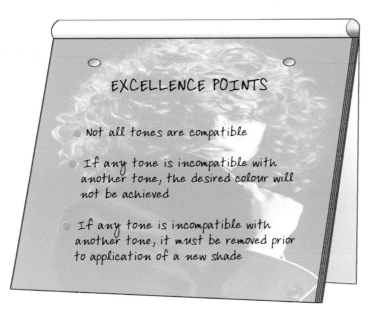

EXCELLENCE POINTS

- Not all tones are compatible

- If any tone is incompatible with another tone, the desired colour will not be achieved

- If any tone is incompatible with another tone, it must be removed prior to application of a new shade

CONTRAINDICATIONS AND THEIR EFFECT ON COLOUR CORRECTION

The following conditions would prevent colour correction taking place:

- The presence of contagious or infectious conditions of the hair and scalp such as ringworm or head lice; refer your client to their GP for medical advice.

- If the hair has poor elasticity or high porosity, it is not advisable to apply a chemical treatment onto damaged hair

- If any incompatible chemicals have been used on the hair, for example products containing metallic salts, which would result in possible further damage to the hair and an unsatisfactory colour result.

- If the client shows a positive reaction to a skin allergy test, never carry out a colouring service that involves tint containing para dye. However, in some cases, a temporary or true vegetable colouring product could be used.

- Other known allergies.

- Medical advice or instructions that may prohibit the use of colouring products, resulting in reducing effectiveness of the medication and affecting the colour result.

- If a test cutting shows a poor colour result.

- If the client has skin sensitivities and disorders you may not be able to carry out the service. Colouring or bleaching (pre-lightening) product must not be applied on any open sores or wounds, breaks in the skin surface or inflammation of the skin.

- If there is a build-up of dark hair colour products on the hair, which are not possible to remove.

COLOUR REDUCTION

Colour reducers, also known as decolourants or colour strippers, are a process that removes artificial colour pigment only from the cortex of the hair. The sole purpose of this type of product is to remove colour that has gone too dark. It is hydrogen-based and reduces the large colour molecules into smaller ones, which are then easily removed from the hair. Some brands only take out the artificial tone and will not alter the natural condition of the hair. However, once the dark colour has been removed it will reveal a warm undercoat. This is normal and due to the previous use of the oxidation tint.

Following manufacturers' instructions, apply the solution to the tinted areas using a tint brush or sponge and leave to develop. Depending on the product you are using you can accelerate the process by adding heat, such as putting your client under a warm hood dryer for up to 15 minutes. Check at five-minute intervals to see how the reducer is developing. Once maximum development time is complete shampoo and rinse up to three times to remove as much pigment as possible then apply a weak peroxide solution to the hair. This will detect any artificial pigment left in the hair. If any of the hair darkens again, reapply fresh colour reducer and repeat the process as before. You can make up to three applications on a head at one sitting.

Once enough pigment has been removed, dry the hair to assess for the following colour service. Always be aware of the increased porosity of the hair after this service and choose your target shade wisely.

TIP	
Target shade When conducting these procedures it is important to remain with your client at all times to allow constant monitoring of the development.	

REDUCTION AND OXIDATION

Reduction is a term that describes the addition of hydrogen to a substance. By the addition of hydrogen you are reducing or 'breaking down' the internal structure of the cortex, for example when using a hydrogen-based product to remove permanent colour it will break down and reduce the artificial colour molecules.

Oxidation is a description of the introduction of oxygen into a substance. When using an oxidation-based colour remover it not only 'lifts' the artificial colour pigment but will also affect the natural pigment. This type of product will give the hair an appearance of being bleached: this is because it is a similar product and both contain oxygen. This is the action of the oxygen contained in the product. It cannot isolate artificial pigment from natural pigment.

Which technique would we use if the present colour is too dark?

Present colour too dark ———▶ Colour-out ———▶ Chosen technique = Deep cleanse

If your client has chosen a new colour which is darker than her existing colour then the colour present will need to be lightened. This technique is called 'deep cleanse'. To do this you will need to use a product designed to remove permanent colour pigment which will remove any unwanted tone and depth of colour.

How do I deep cleanse?

To remove depth using L'Oréal Professionnel Efassor:

- Always begin by using the cleansing technique first to search out the stubborn areas (for step by step on cleanse procedure refer to Chapter 4, p. 97).
- In a non-metallic bowl, mix 1 packet of Efassor with 75mls of 20 or 30 Volume L'Oréal Professionnel Cream Oxidant
- Taking fine sections and starting at the back, apply to the darkest areas first
- Protect the root area with cotton wool strips
- Check regularly until the desired undercoat is achieved
- Development time 50 minutes maximum
- Rinse well and gently shampoo
- Lightly dry
- Apply the target shade to the root area
- Add 15mls of warm water to the remaining mixture
- Take through immediately to the lengths and ends
- Develop for 35 minutes.

PRE-CONDITIONING TREATMENTS

Using conditioner on the hair before colouring is still an unusual procedure within the salon. However, it is a very valuable way of getting the hair back into condition before carrying out any colouring procedure. These conditioners are classified as restructuring treatments and penetrating conditioners. The application of a porosity leveller (penetrating or restructuring conditioner) following the manufacturer's guidelines will help to even out porosity of the hair: to strengthen the cortex use a restructuring treatment also following manufacturers' instructions. Shampooing the hair will remove any barriers that could coat the hair, mainly caused by finishing products such as wax, gel and serum.

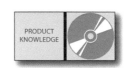

PRODUCT KNOWLEDGE

Pre-pigmentation conditioning treatments and post-colouring conditioning treatments

STEP BY STEP: DEEP CLEANSE

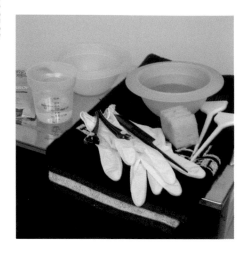

1. Equipment required for gentle cleanse (prior to deep cleanse)

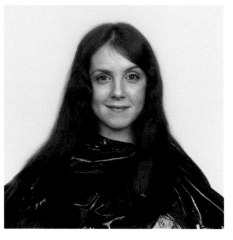

2. Before colour reduction stage 1

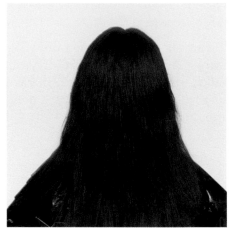

3. Before colour reduction stage 1

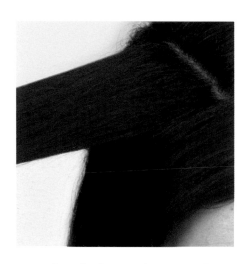

4. Analyse the hair to determine the colour reduction required

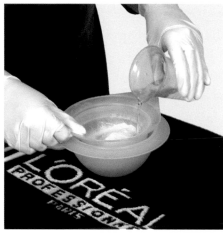

5. Mix product as directed for stage 1

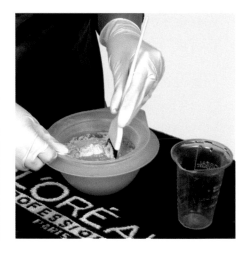

6. Mix product as directed for stage 1

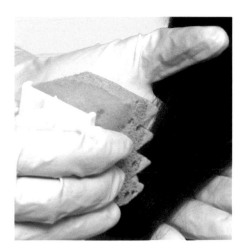

7. Using a sponge, apply product to lengths and ends of the hair

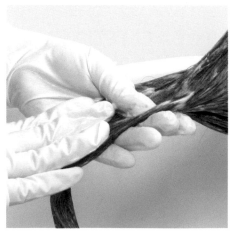

8. Gently massage

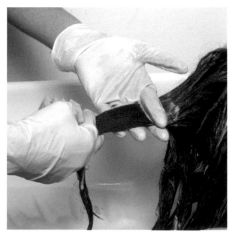

9. Check level of reduction has been achieved

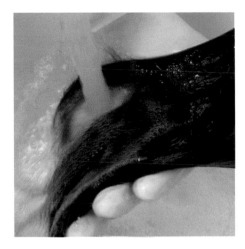

10. Rinse and shampoo

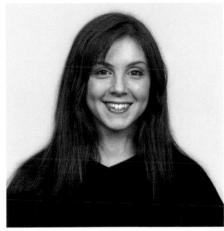

11. Before colour reduction stage 2

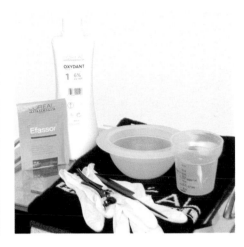

12. Equipment required for deep cleanse

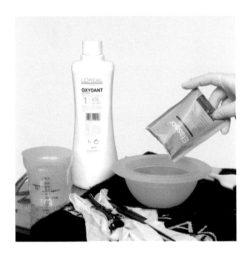

13. Mix products as directed for stage 2

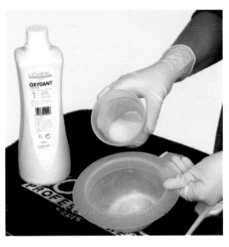

14. Measure required oxidant

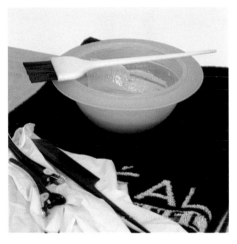

15. Make sure tools are clean for easy application

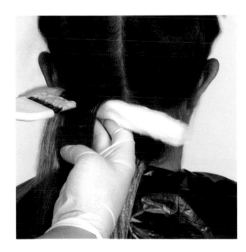

16. Apply reducer to darkest areas

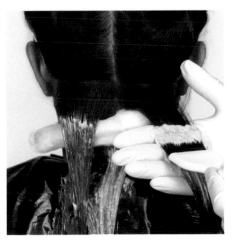

17. Protect natural hair with cotton wool

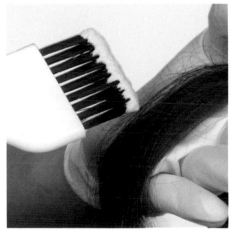

18. Continue application

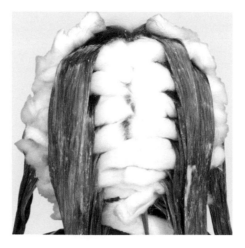

19. Monitor the reduction process

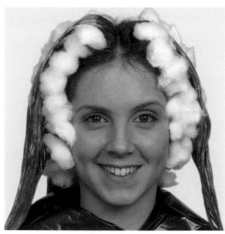

20. Ensure the client is comfortable

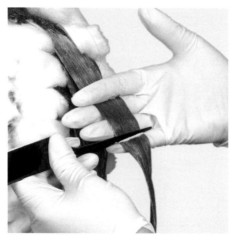

21. Check level of reduction has been achieved

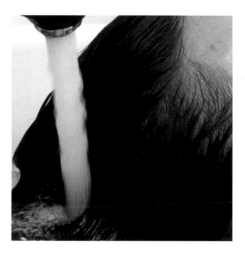

22. Rinse, shampoo and gently dry

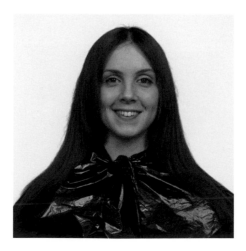

23. Before full head colour application

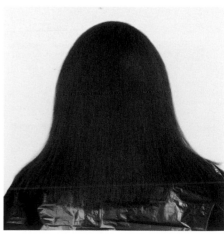

24. Before full head colour application

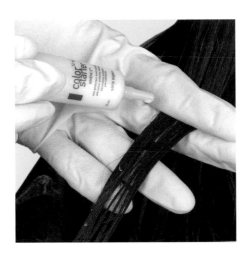

25. Apply porosity leveller to sensitised areas

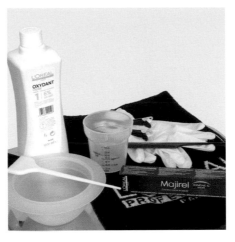

26. Equipment required for full head colour application

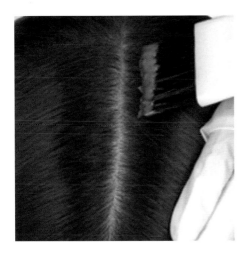

27. Apply chosen shade to the root area

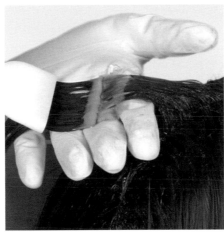

28. Apply to lengths and ends

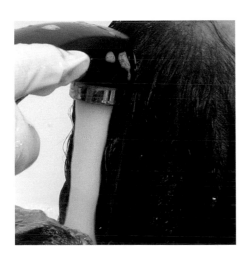

29. Emulsify, rinse and shampoo

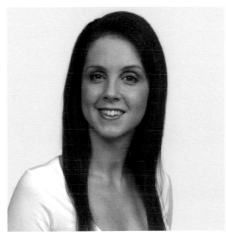

30. Final result

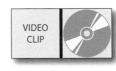

VIDEO CLIP

Steps

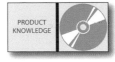

PRODUCT KNOWLEDGE

Product

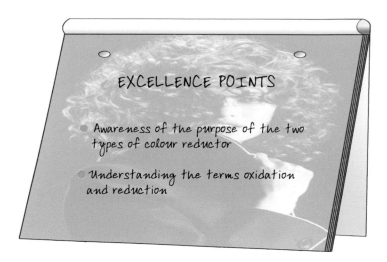

EXCELLENCE POINTS

- Awareness of the purpose of the two types of colour reductor

- Understanding the terms oxidation and reduction

PRE-SOFTENING COLOUR-RESISTANT HAIR

This is carried out before tinting very colour-resistant hair and it will help to ensure good coverage and an even colour result. Coarse resistant hair does tend to be white hair, but this can also occur in fine 'glassy' hair and this is caused by an impacted or tightly closed cuticle (hair that shines like glass). Resistant hair can also be caused by a build up of products. Pre-softening lifts the cuticle of the hair that is resistant to colour, by applying 20 vol (6%) liquid hydrogen peroxide to the resistant areas using a tinting brush.

Pre-soften?

To accommodate a long regrowth or prepare for a virgin head application.

How do we pre-soften?

- Use 20 or 30 volume liquid oxidant
- Apply 1 cm away from scalp
- Dry in to the hair using a warm hand-dryer
- Apply desired target shade
- Take through immediately to lengths and ends
- Develop colour for 35 minutes or according to the manufacturer's instructions
- Always wear protective equipment.

COLOUR-IN – PRE-PIGMENTATION (PRE-COLOUR)

This is a colour replacement technique; it restores depth and tone where colour is missing.

Case study

For example, Olivia has just returned from a holiday in the sun four weeks ago and her hair has lightened. Now her tan has faded her hair colour does not look so good. She would like a new darker colour this time. Her existing colour looks like an 8,34 (light golden copper blonde) and she would like to change to a 6,34 (dark golden copper blonde); this is a common example that you will come across in the salon.

So the existing undercoat which is yellow is too light to support Olivia's chosen shade of 6,34.

Level of lightening	Undercoats
10 – Lightest blonde	Very pale yellow
9 – Very light blonde	Pale yellow
8 – Light blonde	Yellow
7 – Blonde	Yellow orange
6 – Dark blonde	Orange
5 – Light brown	Orange red
4 – Brown	Red
3 – Dark brown	Red
2 – Darkest brown	Red
1 – Black	Red

Therefore, her present shade is a 8,34 and her undercoat is yellow.

Her future dream shade is a 6,34 and an undercoat of orange.

How many levels do we need to darken?

Answer –2 levels

Examples

Present colour	Future colour	Future undercoat
6,34	4,56	Red
9,03	7,4	Yellow orange
8,1	6,34	Orange (incompatible tone)
7,4	5,52	Orange red
10,1	8,34	Yellow (incompatible tone)
9,13	5,35	Orange red (incompatible tone)

Always remember that even though you are going darker with the colour the principle of compatibility of tone is still relevant.

We now know that we must replace the undercoat in Olivia's hair to support the 6,34 shade to obtain the perfect future shade. How do we do this?

There are two ways of replacing a missing undercoat. It depends on:

1 The level of fade in the hair
2 The degree of sensitivity.

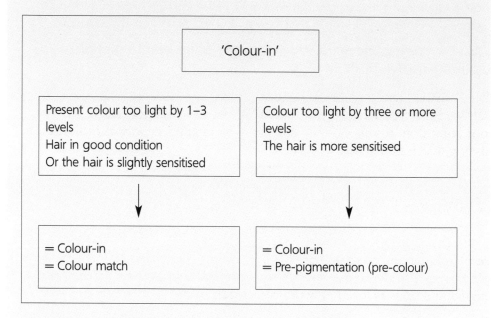

First, let us imagine that Olivia's hair is in relatively good condition. We still have to replace the undercoat by two levels in order to achieve the correct colour.

We need therefore to adapt the technique of colour match to match the lengths and ends by adding the missing undercoat.

WHY COLOUR MATCH?

To match the lengths and ends by adding the missing undercoat.

Colour match is suitable for hair which is faded one, two or three levels and the hair is in good condition or slightly sensitised.

How do I colour match?

- Apply the desired shade to the roots
- Choose a colour match shade that corresponds to the level of the desired shade
- Add 3–6 cm of this shade to the remaining mix
- Add 5–15 mls warm water
- Take through immediately to the lengths and ends
- Develop for 35 minutes.

For example the colour match chart for Majirel is as follows:

Depth of desired shade	Colour match shade
9	8,30
8	8,30
7	7,43–7,45*–7,64*
6	6,45–6,46–6,64*
5	5,4–5,64*
4	4,45–4,56–4,65*

*Majirouge shades

Colour matching is a commercial technique that is used often in the salon. I am sure that you have all seen clients whose hair is highly faded and in poor condition. In this case we need to look at another way of replacing the missing depth undercoat.

WHY PRE-PIGMENT?

Pre-pigmentation (pre-colouring) simply means that instead of adding the colour match shade to the remaining mix, it is applied to the sensitised lengths and ends before applying the desired shade.

These techniques are used when the lengths and ends are three or more levels too light and the hair is sensitised.

How to pre-pigment?

To pre-pigment using L'Oréal Professionnel Majirel:

- Choose a pre-pigmentation (pre-colour) shade which corresponds to the desired shade
- Squeeze 10 cm of the shade into a non-metallic bowl
- Add 15 mls water
- Apply a fine coat of product to the sensitised areas
- **Do not rinse**
- Apply the desired shade to the root area
- Take through immediately to the lengths and ends
- Develop for 35 minutes.

Pre-pigmentation with Majirel

Depth of desired shade	Pre-pigment shade
9	8.30
8	8.30
7	7.43–7.45*–7.64*
6	6.45–6.46–6.64*
5	5.4–5.64*
4	4.45–4.56–4.65*

HOW TO PRE-PIGMENT

To pre-pigment using L'Oréal Professionnel Diacolor Gelée:

- Choose a pre-colour shade which corresponds to the level of the desired shade
- Apply pre-colour mixture to dry hair
- Develop for 15 minutes
- Emulsify and rinse thoroughly
- Apply the desired shade to the roots
- Add 5–15 mls warm water
- Take through immediately to the lengths and ends
- Develop for 35 minutes.

Pre-pigmentation with Diacolour Gelée

Depth	Cool	Warm
9	35 mls gold	
8	20 mls light blonde + 15 mls gold	
7	20 mls blonde + 15 mls gold	20 mls blonde + 15 mls copper
6	20 mls dark blonde + 15 mls gold	20 mls dark blonde + 15 mls copper
5	20 mls light brown + 15 mls gold	20 mls light brown + 15 mls copper
4	20 mls light brown + 15 mls copper	

Always be very methodical and neat with your sectioning technique when applying your colouring product as this will ensure even coverage. Comb through during development, checking that all sections have been evenly covered, and apply more product if needed.

Undercoat pigment + Artificial pigment = Final result

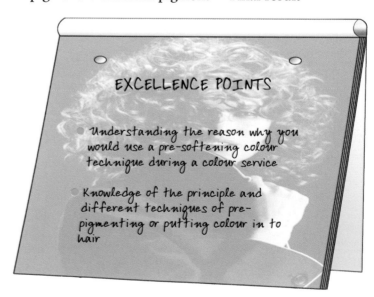

EXCELLENCE POINTS

- Understanding the reason why you would use a pre-softening colour technique during a colour service

- Knowledge of the principle and different techniques of pre-pigmenting or putting colour in to hair

STEP BY STEP: PRE-PIGMENTATION

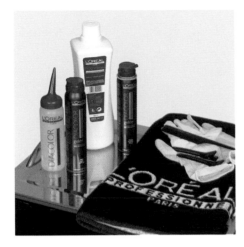

1. Equipment required for pre-pigmentation

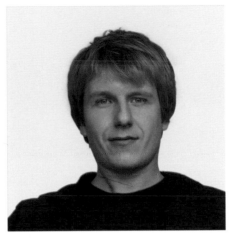

2. Before colour application

TIP

When going darker, sensitised areas of the hair may need a porosity leveller.

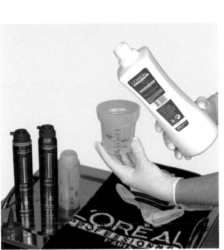

3. Mix product as directed

4. Measure required oxidant

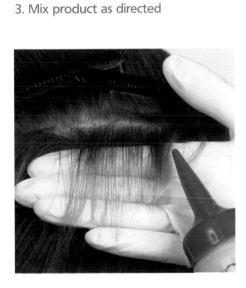

5. Apply chosen pre-pigment to light areas

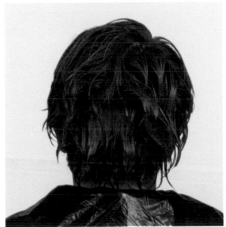

6. Leave for full development time

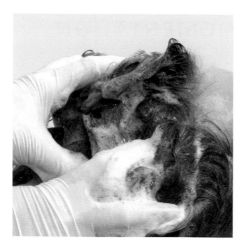

7. Emulsify, rinse and shampoo

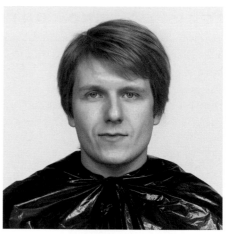

8. After the pre-pigmentation

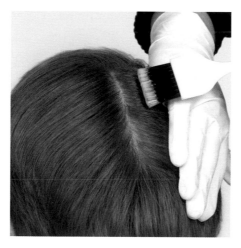

9. Apply chosen shade to regrowth

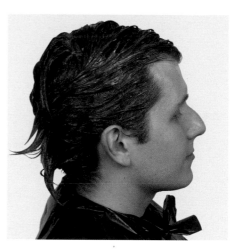

10. Apply to lengths and ends

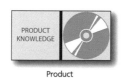

Product

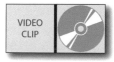

Steps

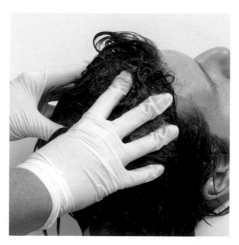

11. Emulsify, rinse and shampoo

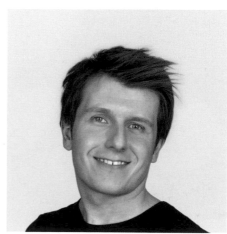

12. Final result

Post-colouring conditioning treatments

The pH of colouring products range from 8–9.5, so always use a pH-balanced conditioner on the hair after every colouring treatment to restore the natural pH of 4.5–5.5 to the hair. The benefits of using a pH balancer are that it closes the cuticle, restores the pH balance to the hair and will help to prevent moisture loss and colour fade.

TIP

Barriers on the hair
Before carrying out a colour correction, you must make sure there are no barriers on the hair i.e. build-up of products such as serum, wax, that could prevent an even result. Use shampoo on the hair to remove these potential barriers: if the build-up is particularly bad massage shampoo onto dry hair then rinse and repeat.

TIP

Manufacturers' instructions
Always read manufacturers' instructions when using these products as they can differ greatly.

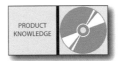
PRODUCT KNOWLEDGE

Pre-pigmentation conditioning treatments and post-colouring conditioning treatments

TIP

pH values of different colouring products

	Approximate value
Stabilised hydrogen peroxide	4
Temporary colour	4–5
Semi-permanent colour	8
Quasi (tone on tone) and permanent colour	9
Bleach (pre-lightener)	8–9.5

Example of ratio of water to hydrogen peroxide to achieve different percentages/volumes.

Start with	Dilute to	Answer
12%	3%	3:1–3 parts water to 1 part 12%
18%	6%	2:1–2 parts water to 1 part 18%
12%	9%	1:3–1 part water to 3 parts 12%

This method will only be accurate with liquid peroxide.
Note: Refer to manufacturer's instructions at all times.

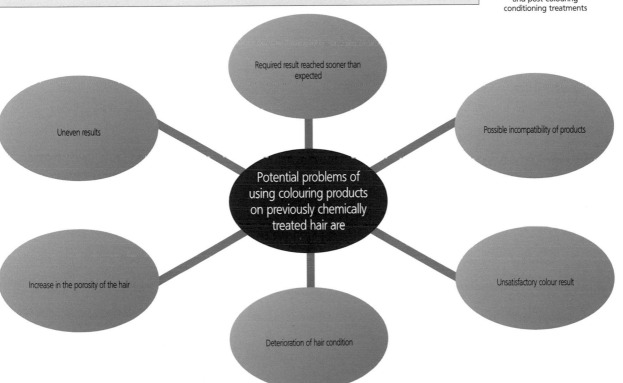

Potential problems of using colouring products on previously chemically treated hair are

- Required result reached sooner than expected
- Possible incompatibility of products
- Unsatisfactory colour result
- Deterioration of hair condition
- Increase in the porosity of the hair
- Uneven results

COLOURING, BLEACHING (PRE-LIGHTENING) AND LIGHTENING TROUBLESHOOTING

The following are common problems that you may encounter, their cause and the remedial action needed.

Problem	Cause	Troubleshooting
Over-processing	• Product left on too long	• Remove product and apply restructurant
	• Hydrogen peroxide too strong	
	• Wrong product used	• Reassess the requirements and apply correct product if condition of hair allows
	• Porous hair	• Advise programme of restructuring treatments prior to further colour or lightening applications
	• Too much heat applied	
Under-processing	• Product not left on long enough	• Reapply and allow full development time
	• Hydrogen peroxide too weak	• Reapply with appropriate strength
	• Not enough product applied	• Reapply with sufficient product if hair condition allows
	• Previous product build-up on hair	• Remove previous product build-up and reapply target product
Skin staining	• Too much product applied	• Remove using stain remover
	• Poor application	
	• Failure to protect the skin	
	• Ineffective removal	
Deterioration of hair condition	• Colouring product too strong	• Use penetrating conditioning treatments
	• Over-processing	
	• Hydrogen peroxide too strong	
	• Too much heat applied	
	• Wrong product used	
Scalp sensitivity	• Hydrogen peroxide too strong	• Remove immediately with tepid water and seek medical advice
	• Bleach or lightening product too strong	
	• Allergic reaction to products	
	• Too much heat applied	• Remove heat source
Product seepage	• Too much product applied	• Recolour affected areas
	• Packet not secure	
	• Prelightener mixture too runny	

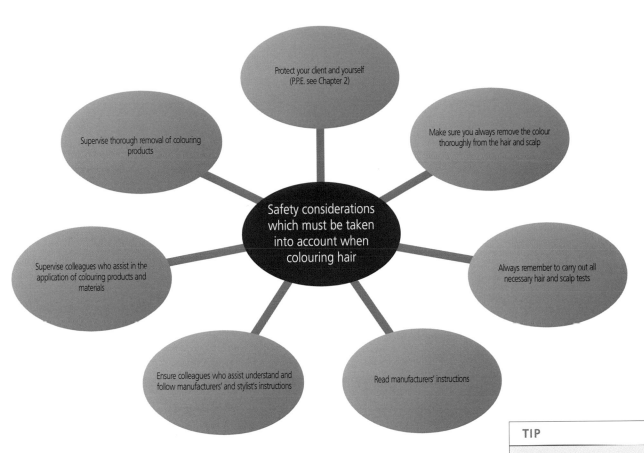

The diagram shows the central topic "Safety considerations which must be taken into account when colouring hair" connected to:
- Protect your client and yourself (P.P.E. see Chapter 2)
- Make sure you always remove the colour thoroughly from the hair and scalp
- Always remember to carry out all necessary hair and scalp tests
- Read manufacturers' instructions
- Ensure colleagues who assist understand and follow manufacturers' and stylist's instructions
- Supervise colleagues who assist in the application of colouring products and materials
- Supervise thorough removal of colouring products

EXCELLENCE POINTS

- The ability to recognise and resolve any colouring problems that you come across

- Knowledge of what safety considerations must be taken into account when colouring hair

Mentoring

When you are working with a colleague who has less technical knowledge and experience than you and they are shadowing you to experience a colour correction procedure, always give clear instructions using a style of language that can be understood, but do not be condescending. Speak clearly in a tone and pitch appropriate to the audience and break down the instructions into small manageable steps. Check to see if your colleague has understood the instructions by asking questions and repeat the instructions if necessary.

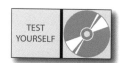

TEST
YOURSELF

Testing and essential
knowledge

Assessment of knowledge and understanding

Test yourself on the content of this chapter by answering these questions. This will help you to prepare for your Essential knowledge/Written test.

1 What details should be included on a client's record card, and when would you complete it?

2 Describe how and why you would:
   (a) Pre-soften hair
   (b) Pre-pigment (pre-colour) hair.

3 Why is it important to restore the hair's natural pH after a colouring and bleaching service?

4 How can contra-indications affect the delivery of a colour correction service?

5 Why is it important to section the hair accurately during a colour service?

6 State three reasons why it is important to record test results.

7 Describe the principles of colour selection by:
   (a) Drawing a diagram of the colour wheel
   (b) Stating the three primary colours
   (c) Identifying the colours that neutralise each of the primary colours
   (d) What is the purpose of the International Colour Code?

8 Complete the table below stating why we should use pre-pigmentation and post-colouring treatments on the hair before and after carrying out any colouring or lightening services.

	How	Why
Pre-pigmentation conditioning treatments	•	•
	•	•
Post-colouring conditioning treatments	•	•
	•	•

9 Describe four ways of giving clear instructions to a colleague with less experience than yourself.

10 When questioning clients to establish if they have any contra-indications describe:
    (a) Why it is important to question the client
    (b) Why it is important to document the clients' responses
    (c) What is the legal significance of questioning and recording their responses?

11 State three reasons why it is important to follow the manufacturer's instructions for skin allergy testing.

12 Outline the principles of colour correction.

13 What do the terms 'oxidation' and 'reduction' mean?

14 Work out the different ratios needed for the required hydrogen peroxide strength.

Start with	Dilute to	Answer
12%	3%	
18%	6%	
12%	9%	

15 What are the pH values of the following products:
   (a) Stabilised hydrogen peroxide
   (b) Temporary colour
   (c) Semi-permanent colour
   (d) Quasi (tone on tone) and permanent colour
   (e) Bleach.

16 When would you use different methods of colour removers to remove artificial colour? Include the methods for applying and removing in your answer.

17 For each of the following colouring, lightening and bleaching problems, state:
   (a) The cause
   (b) The remedial action you would take
       – Over-processing
       – Under-processing
       – Skin staining
       – Deterioration of hair condition
       – Scalp sensitivity
       – Product seepage.

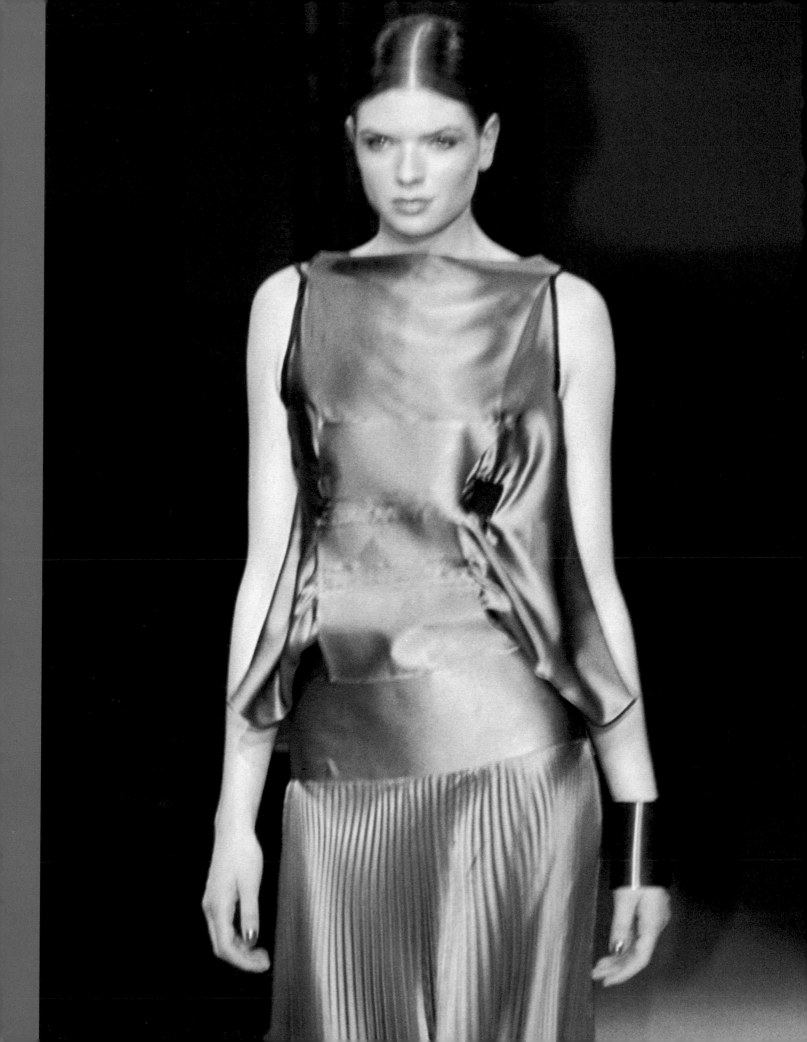

The client journey

If you're reading this and you don't care about people, move on to another career.

Michelle Blake, Style Consultant, Blushes

'They come in, ask questions, and want to know the prices', snapped the shop owner. We can assume she wasn't the star of the customer service seminar. She may even be entitled to a refund.

For Michelle Blake, style consultant at Blushes, consultation is the key to success. Try to set aside fifteen to twenty minutes for consultation, and if possible, ask the client to come in prior to the appointment, especially with a new customer. As the colourist, you don't necessarily need to do the consultation, but make sure everything is kept on record.

Try to understand the personality of your client. Will an elegant, high-maintenance look work on someone who's very casual? They may not know what's involved. Even with regular customers, a prior consultation can help to refresh or refine what they usually have. If they want something you feel is unsuitable, don't be negative. Find out what they like about what they're asking for, and offer an alternative.

Remember that what may seem like small points can make a difference. Sit down with the client, make eye contact, and don't touch the hair too soon – it means you've stopped listening.

With so much competition around, good consultation, good communication and good manners can make the difference between one visit and a regular customer.

chapter 5

THE CLIENT JOURNEY

Learning objectives

In this chapter, you will gain the skills you need to communicate effectively when consulting with your clients and learn how to offer professional help and guidance when appropriate throughout their salon experience. In *the client journey*, we will consider:

- **The perfect client journey**
- **Verbal and non-verbal communication**
- **Working as a team**
- **Consulting with your clients**
- **Identifying your client's needs and wishes**
- **Open and closed questioning techniques**
- **Pre-treatment testing**
- **Adverse hair and scalp conditions**
- **Describing the features and benefits to your client**
- **Treatment timings**
- **Ranges of treatments and their costs**
- **Location, location, location!**
- **Promote additional products or treatments to clients**
- **Top tips for recommendations**
- **Top tips for merchandising**
- **Salon legal requirements**

G6 Promote additional products or services to clients

G7 Advise and consult with clients

G9 Provide hairdressing consultation services

G11 Contribute to the financial effectiveness of the business

The client journey

Client journey

Follow the client journey and see the opportunities to recommend retail with your clients and expose them to products

Advise, discuss, recommend – you don't have to sell

10.30am
Client arrives

10.30am–10.40am
Waiting area

Place the retail stand nearby with good product information to allow client to browse

10.40am–10.50am
Consultation

Advise on a treatment before going to the backwash. Talk about hair care needs with the client

10.50am–11am
At the backwash

Use backwash sizes of retail products. The fantastic smell and feel of the hair after washing promote interest in the products used. Display backwash neatly and clearly for the client to see

11am–12pm
Styling unit

Place retail sizes of the backwash product used on the styling unit. Display retail promotional material for the client to read. Place magazines to read with product features highlighted. Discuss styling products used on the client

12pm–12.10pm
Reception

A great time to inspire an impulse purchase – just like the chocolate at the supermarket check-out! Create a fantastic display here with your mini stocker unit

VERBAL AND NON-VERBAL COMMUNICATION

Verbal and non-verbal communication can be demonstrated in many ways. To communicate effectively with your clients, you will need to be fluent in both. Effective communication with your clients and colleagues ensures that accurate information is given and obtained. Promoting good relationships between clients and salon staff presents a professional salon image and creates a good foundation for a successful business.

Verbal communication

As a hairdresser, you will need to be good at communicating verbally with your clients and also your colleagues. You will need to be skilled at using talk as a medium to understand your client's requirements and also when working as part of a team.

Verbal communication should be carried out:

- Clearly
- Confidently
- Honestly
- Politely
- Tactfully
- In a responsive manner.

Examples of verbal communication may include:

- Speaking with someone face-to-face
- Making an appointment over the telephone
- Consulting with your clients prior to an appointment.

Non-verbal communication

Your professionalism is transferred to your clients within thirty seconds of them first seeing you – this is known as non-verbal communication. Remember that the way we present ourselves can and does affect how a client will respond to us.

To communicate non-verbally:

- Use eye contact
- Have friendly facial expressions
- Maintain an open and relaxed manner
- Present a professional appearance.

Examples of non-verbal communications may include:

- Writing down a message
- Recording an appointment
- Reading and/or writing a letter
- Gestures
- Sign language
- Body language (positive and negative).

Working as a team

A bad atmosphere in a salon between staff can be due to poor communication between colleagues. If this is not addressed, confrontation situations could occur leading to a possible breach of confidentiality. Gossiping to clients about your colleagues is *very* unprofessional and this in turn could result in a warning or possible termination of your contract with the salon, loss of salon business, loss of goodwill with your clientele and possibly a bad reputation.

Learn how to use varied tones of speech and use your body language positively when dealing with clients and colleagues. Communication is about expressing your ideas or opinions in a positive manner. To present a positive discussion, you must exchange information.

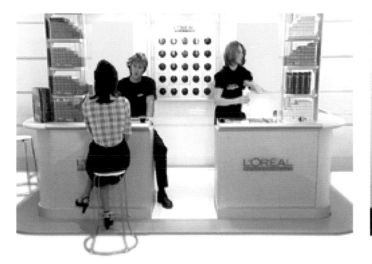

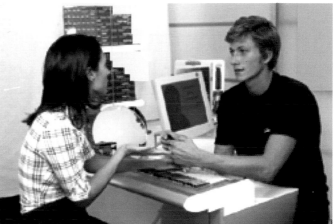

You will need to be good at both verbal and non-verbal communication

---

ACTIVITY

Verbal and non-verbal communication
Think of behaviour that you can adopt to encourage others to communicate. Role play with a colleague creating a simple dialogue of a professional conversation. Take it in turns to convey your verbal and non-verbal communication both negatively and positively.

Communication signals

Vary the way in which you speak; not all clients can be spoken to in the same way. Learn to move the conversation forward by developing points and ideas, remembering to focus on the purpose of the discussion.

Show the client that you are listening by varying your body language, listening closely and sensitively. Learn how to respond appropriately by asking questions to show an interest in what the client is saying. This will come with experience and as soon as you start to consult with clients, you will begin to develop your communication skills.

Clients may be in a hurry and not have enough time to talk, other than to make an appointment. They may be here in reception to complain or make a comment about a particular aspect of the business. Their tone of voice, delivery and speed of speech, body language, manner, vocabulary and facial expression will tell you how that client is feeling.

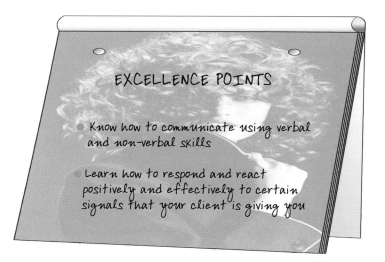

EXCELLENCE POINTS

● Know how to communicate using verbal and non-verbal skills

● Learn how to respond and react positively and effectively to certain signals that your client is giving you

---

ACTIVITY

Client feelings
Role play with a colleague; vary your vocabulary, body language and listening skills in various salon situations. Salon situations may be busy, quiet, your client may be angry, nervous and shy or you or your client may be feeling ill. Think of a few more situations to demonstrate the ways that you would deal with clients.

CONSULTING WITH YOUR CLIENTS

The purpose of consulting with your clients is to make sure:

- The client's hair and scalp is suitable for the requested treatment
- The most suitable products, tools and equipment are used
- The most suitable techniques for creating the desired effect and look are agreed and used
- The client's needs and wishes are met
- Additional products and techniques are recommended to the client
- The client's lifestyle is discussed briefly to determine if your client can maintain their hair at home.

Begin by greeting your clients in a manner appropriate to their needs: they may be elderly, use a walking stick, or even need some assistance with salon doors when bringing a pushchair, pram or buggy into the salon. You will then need to communicate well in your consultation and be effective in your analysis of that consultation.

- **Consultation**: Seeking information about your client and what they would like to happen to their hair
- **Analysis**: to examine, and as a result of this examination identify any disease or disorder which may indicate that it is not safe to proceed with the treatment, or to make suitable recommendations for conditions of the hair and scalp that the professional stylist can treat.

Identifying your client's needs and wishes

Staff need sufficient time to discuss what is best for their clients' hair and scalp. Using a consultation card or sheet will help you work through all of the stages necessary.

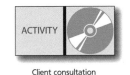

ACTIVITY

Client consultation

> **ACTIVITY**
>
> **Furthering the conversation**
> Think of three ways that you can move the client conversation forward.

> **TIP** ✔
>
> Ideally, both you and your client should be seated throughout the consultation. Imagine how you would feel if you were seated and the person speaking to you was standing over you – this often gives an impression of intimidation. If you are both seated it will help to ensure positive eye contact between client and stylist and will give your client confidence that they are receiving professional advice and guidance. Remember that it is your job to make sure that your client feels respected and welcome in your salon.

OPEN AND CLOSED QUESTIONS

Talking to a client when you are a hairdresser should never be a problem as we tend to be natural communicators. However, you must learn to use the correct kind of questions – we call these open and closed questions. Asking appropriate and relevant questions in a way your client will understand encourages them to speak about their hair.

First, open up the consultation by letting your client tell you how she is feeling about her hair, for example 'How do you feel about your hair?'. Some people can articulate clearly exactly what their requirements are, and you will have no problem in establishing a plan of action. However, other people are not at their most confident within the salon atmosphere and even feel a little intimidated. They sometimes feel too shy to tell you exactly what they require. The use of open questions will help to encourage the client to tell you any information that you require to perform a satisfactory colouring service on their hair.

Open questions

If you need information from your client use questions that begin with Who, How, What, Where, Would and When: these will lead to more information than a question that can be answered with 'Yes' or 'No'.

For example:

- *'How would you like to have your hair coloured today?'*
  This is a good basic opener to lead your client into stating exactly what she would like the colour result to be.
- *'What tone do you prefer, gold or ash?'*
  This again leads you to a better understanding of your client's requirements.
- *'Would you like to look at the shade chart and tell me what your likes/dislikes are?'*
  The shade chart is also a good communication tool and icebreaker which helps the client to feel more in control of what she is having done with her hair because she can start to visualise her dream colour.

Encourage your client to ask about areas they are unsure of and confirm your understanding of her wishes with her before making any recommendations.

Closed questions

These types of questions will only give you one-word answers and limit the amount of information provided to you by the client. Use these types of questions when you need a definite 'Yes' or 'No'. They are very useful but really only needed when you are repeating back to your client your understanding of what she requires.

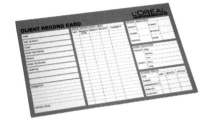

Always record details of consultations on the client's record card

For example:

- *'So we are going to lighten your hair by two shades today?'*
- *'And you want a gold tone as opposed to an ash?'*

Confirm your client's treatment by repeating the information; record it on the client's record card when the treatment is complete.

For more information on questioning techniques, please refer to Chapter 4, Colour change, P. 84.

ACTIVITY

Ask six clients the following questions and compare the amount and type of information you have received. What type of question received the most information from the client?

- Do you style your own hair?
- How do you style your hair at home?
- How often do you have your haircut?
- How do you like your haircut?
- What do you like about your hair?
- Do you have any limitations with your treatment today?

FIRST IMPRESSIONS

Seat your client comfortably in a quiet area, usually in the reception. Make sure that you are at the same level as your client and begin your consultation.

First impressions make a lasting impression. When we first meet our client, we have about ten seconds from the first eye contact to convey the correct professional image. The client in turn will also analyse what they see: therefore it is important that our appearance is as professional as it possibly can be. Take into account that not all clients or even indeed all salon owners will welcome bare midriffs, tattooed navels, body or facial piercing, or sleeveless tops. Remember that a consultation should be as professional and as discreet as you can make it. First impressions *do* count.

Identify and confirm the needs of your clients and always treat them courteously, even when working under pressure. Look out for signs that your client may need you or want something from you.

Clients with special requirements

Use discretion and tact when dealing with those clients who have a particular need such as a sight or hearing difficulty. Learn how to adapt to their requirements and respond positively to their requests. Make the best possible use of your time by asking relevant questions. Demonstrate to your client that you are interested in them and their hair; this will make for a more efficient service and makes the best possible use of both stylist and client time. Remember that your tone of voice should remain calm and even, and respond by using positive and appropriate body language.

Focus on the main point of the comment that the client is making and move the conversation to a satisfactory conclusion. Develop the important points of the conversation, focus on the purpose and summarise the client's comments to clarify the situation. Vary how and when to participate in the client's discussion: often you can pick up a great deal by listening to what the client is saying, but read between the lines by observing their body language.

Remember that your clients' opinion of how professional your salon is will depend on the behaviour of everybody within the salon.

> **TIP**
>
> Clients will enjoy the experience of good client care so remember to communicate and give them a positive impression of you and the salon at all times. Clients will not notice potential problems if you are dealing with them calmly as they arise. Do not let yourself or the salon down by expressing negative facial expressions. Your level of professionalism must remain consistent for new and returning clients at all times.

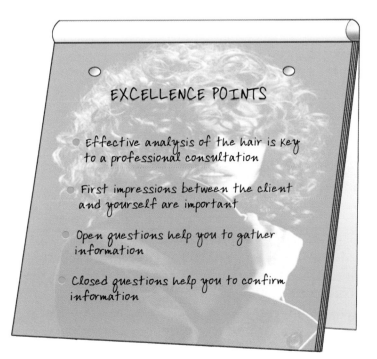

EXCELLENCE POINTS

- Effective analysis of the hair is key to a professional consultation

- First impressions between the client and yourself are important

- Open questions help you to gather information

- Closed questions help you to confirm information

TIP

Be careful not to choose too warm a colour if your client has naturally red cheeks.

Skin tone

Skin tone is an important factor to consider as part of your consultation. Your clients may be Asian, African-Caribbean or European, so you will encounter a varied range of skin tones. Many British Europeans have a pale skin tone compared with other nationalities which may be olive in tone, darker in colour or with natural rosy cheeks. Together with the colour of your client's eyes, current hairstyle and clothes that they wear, this makes for a super foundation on which to build your colour consultation.

Suitable topics of conversation

TIP

Not all clients like to talk about themselves and may prefer to ask you about yourself instead, but do be careful not to talk too much about yourself. It may be that the client is interested in your weekend, your recent holiday or your plans for your next weekend, but don't assume that your colleagues will be if they have heard the finer details three times already that morning!

Remember the client is the reason that you are there; you must demonstrate a professional and business-like approach to all aspects of the client's visit. Conduct also features within your personal presentation; all that you say and do is part of you as a professional person. It is pointless being correctly dressed only to follow it through with inappropriate conversation and conduct.

You will need to use your communication skills to work out where your client would like the conversation to go. Often, a client's visit to the salon will be a rare opportunity to enjoy some personal time away from the stresses and strains of their everyday life. They may welcome the opportunity to forget about work, the family and everything else they usually find occupies their mind and enjoy some trivial chit-chat with you. They may also like to talk about themselves: to feel that they are the most important issue to be discussed for a change!

TIP

Conversations about personal issues such as sex, drugs, religion and politics can cause friction within the salon and are best avoided.

HEALTH AND SAFETY

Manufacturer's instructions
Clients place themselves in your expert hands, and expect an extremely professional treatment. You are bound by the manufacturer's instructions to carry out hair and skin allergy tests to prevent damage to the client's hair and skin.

HAIR AND SKIN ALLERGY TESTS

Most of the tests involved prior to colouring only take a few minutes during consultation; the long-term benefits are that the client's hair is assessed correctly prior to the colouring service. The results of the tests will give both stylist and client a better and more accurate understanding what the actual result will be, giving both parties the opportunity to reconsider their options if necessary.

ACTIVITY

Look at the table below and complete the table by answering each question linked to the hair sensitivity or skin allergy test.

When, why and how do you carry out each of the necessary tests?

What will the outcomes be?

Incompatibility test	Porosity test	Elasticity test	Strand test	Skin test
How	How	How	How	How
When	When	When	When	When
Why	Why	Why	Why	Why

TIP

All manufacturers' instructions will recommend a skin allergy test prior to colouring the client's hair. This is a standard professional practice and must be carried out before each colouring treatment that touches the scalp. Irrespective of the client having colour applied to the hair and scalp for many years, the skin can change its own natural tolerance to substances on a regular basis.

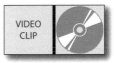

A skin allergy test

Skin allergy test

If the colour product contains paraphenylene diamine (para dye), the skin allergy test *must* be carried out prior to the colour application. The manufacturer's instructions must be read and followed and the test applied 48 hours prior to the colour application. This is essential if the colour product containing para dye is going to be in contact with the scalp.

It is of the utmost importance to inform members of the public about any procedure undertaken that may affect their health and safety. This may involve skin allergy testing prior to the application of quasi (tone on tone) and permanent colours. This can be carried out via the initial client consultation, 48 hours before the colour application.

To see step by step instructions on how to do a skin allergy test, see Chapter 3, P. 52.

Incompatibility test

Metallic salts are incompatible with hydrogen peroxide. These metallic salts can be found in compound organic henna and hair colour restorer for both men and women. The hair may bubble, boil and/or break if metallic salts are present.

The incompatibility test is therefore used to detect chemicals/elements which could react with hairdressing processes such as colouring and perming. The test is carried out as follows:

1 Protect your hands by wearing suitable disposable gloves.

2 Place a small cutting of hair in a small bowl.

3 Pour into the bowl a mixture of 20 parts of 6% hydrogen peroxide and 1 part ammonium thioglycolate (general purpose perm solution). Make sure that you are not bending over the bowl to avoid splashing the chemicals on to your face or inhaling any resultant released fumes.

4 Watch for signs of bubbling, heating or discolouration. These indicate that the hair already contains incompatible chemicals. The hair should not be permed, tinted or bleached (pre-lightened) if there are any signs of reaction. Perming treatments might discolour or break the hair and could burn the skin.

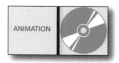

A porosity test

A porosity test

Used prior to shampooing when the hair is dry to identify if the cuticle scales are intact or damaged. This will help clarify the most appropriate product to be used on your client's hair. Remember that a damaged cuticle can absorb products quickly and may lead to colour fade on the porous parts of the hair shaft. Be careful with your colour choice and choice of product.

To see step by step instructions on how to do a porosity test, see Chapter 1.

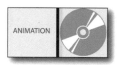

An elasticity test

An elasticity test

This is carried out on wet hair. Wet hair will stretch more readily due to the water molecules stretching and breaking the temporary hydrogen bonds. These hydrogen bonds are rejoined when the hair is styled and dried.

To see step by step instructions on how to do an elasticity test, see Chapter 1.

TIP
Always consult the record card of an existing client to identify any influencing factors that may affect the current or future treatments.

TIP
Hair that is porous and lacks elasticity indicates the need for a gentle approach in terms of choosing a semi-permanent colour instead of a permanent colour, or a high-lift tint instead of bleach (pre-lightener).

Conduct the following hair sensitivity tests following manufacturers' instructions and recognised industry procedures.

HEALTH AND SAFETY
If a client has a positive allergic reaction to a permanent colour, which can range from itchy red sore skin to swelling of the body, they must seek medical help and attention immediately.

Testing	Why would you do this test?	Expected result	When to do the test	Potential consequences of not carrying out the test
Elasticity test	To determine the condition of the cortex	The hair should have enough elasticity (strength) to return to its original length	During consultation and before any colouring service	Damage will occur to the hair
Porosity test	To determine the condition of the cuticle	The hair should feel uneven when felt from ends to roots	During consultation and before any colouring service	
Incompatibility test	To determine the presence of metallic salts	If the hair contains metallic salts, the solution will bubble and become hot, the hair will discolour and start to disintegrate	During consultation and before any colouring service	Hair will disintegrate, change colour causing damage to the hair
Skin allergy test	To test for allergic reaction to colour products	Positive reaction – skin will become red, irritated and sore. It could be itchy, weepy and swollen	48 hours before the application of a permanent tint	Contact dermatitis and in severe cases anaphylactic shock
Strand test	To check the development of colour or bleach (pre-lightening) applications. You would only do this test after prior assessment of the suitability to carry out a colour	To see if the colour result has developed sufficiently to remove	After manufacturer's recommended development time	Colour result unsatisfactory

Suggested courses of action after testing

- **Elasticity test**

  If the hair breaks or remains stretched:

  Do not proceed with any colouring or bleaching service.

  Advise a series of penetrating conditioning or restructuring treatments.

  If the hair returns to normal length:

  Proceed with colouring or bleaching service.

- **Porosity test**

  If the hair feels rough and uneven:

  Carry out test cutting to check for even colour result.

  Apply a pre-pigmentation (pre-colour) conditioner to level out porosity.

  Advise series of conditioning treatments before any colour application.

  If the hair feels smooth and even:

  Proceed with colouring or bleaching service.

- **Incompatibility test**

  If there is no change to hair or liquid:

  Proceed with colouring or bleaching service.

  If you have a slight increase in the temperature of the liquid:

  If the hair changes colour or if the liquid bubbles or fizzes:

  Do not proceed with any colour service.

- **Skin allergy test**

  Positive reaction:

  Do not proceed under any circumstances.

  Negative reaction:

  Proceed with colouring service.

- **Strand test**

  If the hair colour is not the required result:

  Leave colouring product to develop further until required result is achieved.

  If the hair colour is the required result:

  Remove colouring products.

EXCELLENCE POINTS

During consultation, consideration of the client's eye colour and skin tone are important when selecting a suitable colour

Not all topics of conversation are appropriate for discussion with your client

In order to maintain a professional service, carrying out the relevant hair sensitivity and skin allergy tests is essential

Adverse hair and scalp conditions

Internal and external factors relating to hair and scalp condition must be taken into consideration before colouring a client's hair. These factors can affect or limit the services offered to your client.

A client may have:

- oily hair and scalp due to too much sebum being secreted along the hair shaft
- normal, dry or dandruff-affected hair and scalp
- fine, coarse or medium-textured hair
- varying levels of porosity along the hair length
- previous chemical treatments
- cuts or scratches on the scalp
- psoriasis
- eczema
- recent scar tissue
- boils, sebaceous cysts.

The purpose of the hair and scalp analysis is to ensure the treatment is appropriate, effective and safe for a client with any of these conditions.

Infectious disorders and infestations

Hair, skin and scalp conditions have to be considered prior to carrying out any colouring treatment. Problems encountered include infections and or infestations.

As a general rule suspected infestations may be recognised by itchy skin or scalp, the presence of a rash, redness and the presence of the parasite with, possibly, visible eggs. Some important things to remember are:

- A doctor should always treat infections and diseases of the hair and scalp.
- Non-infectious diseases may be treated in the salon or by a trichologist (a hair and scalp specialist).
- Referral to a pharmacist may be necessary if your client has pediculous capitis (head lice).

The following conditions will prevent the colouring or bleaching treatment from being carried out.

Pediculosis capitis is commonly known as head lice and is an infestation by parasites, pediculous humanus corpis are body lice and phthirus pubis refers to the pubic louse. These are very contagious conditions and they must not be treated by the professional stylist. Clients must be referred to a doctor or pharmacist for further treatment.

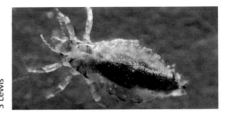

S Lewis

Pediculosis capitis

Scabies is commonly known as the itch mite and is caused by the mite *Sarcoptes Scabiei*. This condition can be recognised by intense itching, particularly at night. Sometimes the burrows that the itch mite makes are visible and are grey in colour with scaly swellings, reddish lumps may appear later. This is a highly contagious condition passed on by close physical contact. The professional stylist must not treat this client and referral to a doctor is necessary.

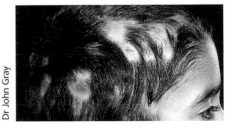

Dr M H Beck

Scabies

Fungal diseases such as **tinea capitis**, which is ringworm of the scalp, is recognised by round bald, sometimes itchy areas on the scalp with broken hair stubble. Tinea is the name given to any fungal condition that may affect the skin, nails and or hair. The skin may be inflamed and can have a musty smell. This is a very infectious condition and must not be treated by the professional stylist. Referral to a doctor is necessary.

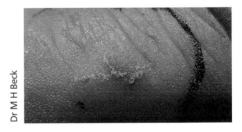

Dr John Gray

Tinea capitis

Impetigo is skin that reddens and has small, fluid-filled blisters. The blisters tend to burst, leaving moist, weeping areas that dry to leave honey-coloured crusts. This is a bacterial infection, usually *Staphylococci* entering broken areas of the skin, and is highly infectious. This condition is sometimes caused by shaving too close and can cause ingrown hairs. The professional stylist should recommend the client consults their doctor for further treatment.

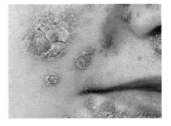

Impetigo

Folliculitis is recognised by pus-filled blisters around the follicle. This inflammation of the hair follicle can affect one or many hair follicles. This is a bacterial infectious condition, usually with the bacteria *Staphylococcus Aureus*. The professional stylist would not carry out any hairdressing treatments and referral to a doctor is necessary.

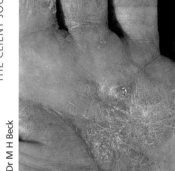

Dr M H Beck

Eczema

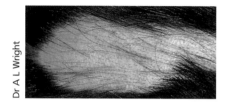

Dr A L Wright

Alopecia

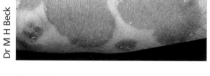

Dr M H Beck

Psoriasis

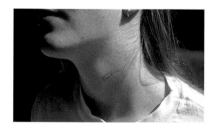

Keloid scar

Non-infectious conditions

Eczema and **dermatitis** is recognised by irritable, localised itching, usually on the hands and in between the fingers, usually due to an allergy. This condition can sometimes be brought on by stress; swelling may occur, together with open, weeping cracks in the skin. Should your client have this condition do not apply any chemicals to open and weeping skin; this would be an unprofessional and negligent act and you may be liable to prosecution.

HEALTH AND SAFETY	

Non-infectious conditions

Dermatitis and eczema are non-infectious conditions and are usually an occupational risk to the practising stylist. Particular care must be taken when dealing with products: *always* rinse and dry your hands *thoroughly*.

Alopecia is a hair loss condition of varying degrees and types. It can be found on any hairy part of the body. It is usually due to male hormones, and is sometimes caused by shock, trauma, childbirth, accident or because of an operation. The western world has the highest percentage of male pattern baldness when compared with its Asian or European neighbours. This is a non-infectious condition. Specialist stylists, trichologists and doctors could treat a client with this condition.

Psoriasis is recognised by the presence of thickened patches of red inflamed skin covered with silvery scales. This inherited condition tends to clear and reoccurs, usually at times of stress. This is a non-infectious condition and it is safe to carry out hairdressing treatments.

Dandruff can be recognised by white flakes on the scalp and through the hair. Dandruff can be dry or oily and is usually attributed to an increased production of epidermal skin cells. This is a non-infectious condition and it is safe to carry out hairdressing treatments.

Keloids are a raised, hard, irregularly-shaped itchy scar on the skin due to a defective healing process in which too much collagen is produced, usually after a skin injury. This condition is usually found in clients who are African-Caribbean. Hairdressing treatments should be considered in terms of how recent tissue scarring is. Always refer the client to a doctor if in any doubt. Always deal promptly and efficiently with analysis of problems as identified by you and/or your colleagues.

Recommendations on the colour service must be based on the outcomes of your hair and scalp analysis. Consider suggestions about alternative treatments and products if you decide your client's requirements are unrealistic. Known allergies and skin disorders must be identified at the consultation stage where any medical advice and or instructions between the client and stylist can be clarified and acted upon.

Give accurate advice on an alternative course of action if your client's preferred treatment is not possible.

DESCRIBING THE FEATURES AND BENEFITS OF PRODUCTS TO YOUR CLIENTS

The features and benefits of any product or treatment must be fairly and legally described. It is your responsibility to make it clear to all visitors, staff and clients that the products and treatments available in your salon are of a merchantable quality. The Trade Descriptions Act 1968 and 1972 states quite clearly 'that products should not be falsely or misleadingly described in relation to its quality, fitness, price or purpose, by advertisements, orally, displays or descriptions'. Think about using a variety of products as you colour, cut and style the clients hair. Use the actual bottle or jar of product to better explain the features and benefits of the product, how to apply and what to expect as an end result. Make sure that you explain how to use the product in accordance with the manufacturer's instructions and be careful not to claim that the product will do something that it is not supposed to do. Explore the various looks possible with your client by using relevant visual aids.

- A feature of a colour treatment is what it does and how it will look on the client, such as highlights to emphasis the shape of the cut.

- The benefit is what that means to the client and the hairdresser.

ACTIVITY

Client records

Many salons have now adopted various software and hardware equipment to assist them in their daily business. This could include making client appointments, stock checks, calculating commission, salaries and keeping client details on a database. Discuss with a colleague the advantages of carrying out and completing a consultation sheet.

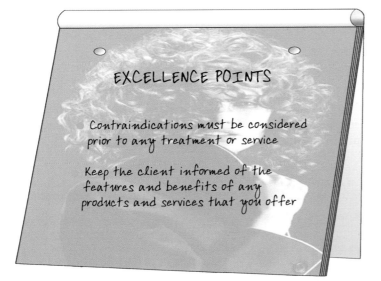

EXCELLENCE POINTS

Contraindications must be considered prior to any treatment or service

Keep the client informed of the features and benefits of any products and services that you offer

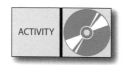

ACTIVITY

How long should a
colouring service take me?

TREATMENT TIMINGS

It is particularly good practice to discuss the whole treatment at the consultation stage, including the likely duration and what the client can expect during the visit. Consider explaining how long each stage of the treatment will take, the cost involved and any necessary products that will enhance the life of the colour on the client's hair. Once you have agreed the treatments with your client make a suitable appointment for the agreed services.

Some specialised treatments may take longer than the usual salon treatment your client receives and this must be made clear to your client at the time of making the appointment. Your client's comfort may be affected by the length of time that they are in the salon and they may have to make special dietary arrangements or find someone to pick up a child from school. It is reasonable to expect that your clients also have busy lives and it is good business sense to give them an indication of the approximate time involved.

Realistic times for colour and bleach within a commercial salon

Mix and apply colour for a full head permanent colour	45 mins
Mix and apply colour for a regrowth permanent colour	25 mins
Mix and apply bleach for a full head bleach	45 mins
Pull through highlights/lowlights to include preparation and application for a full head	35 mins
Woven highlights/lowlights to include preparation and application for a full head	45/60 mins
Block colour partial head	45/60 mins
Colour correction	60 mins
Coloured hair extensions (each extension)	10/15 mins
Temporary coloured hair mascara	10/15 mins

All staff must be fully conversant with the treatments, cost and products on offer within the salon. Effective communication will ensure that accurate information is given and obtained. This leads to a good relationship with clients and promotes a professional image for the salon and its staff.

TIP

If the cost is discussed when making an appointment over the telephone, be sure to use the word *'from'* when quoting the cost of a treatment, e.g. *'from'* £25. This will prevent any future discrepancy or argument when the client comes to the salon to have their hair coloured.

THE RANGE OF TREATMENTS AND HOW MUCH THEY COST

Technical treatments available in your salon may range from cuts, colours, and perms; finishes could include blow drying, finger drying and setting. The cost of each treatment offered within the salon will depend on various factors.

There may be a scale of costs for each treatment dependent on who actually carries out the treatment. A junior member of staff may charge less than a senior member of staff. This must be made clear to the client at the time of booking the appointment and clarified at the time of consultation.

Some salons ask for a deposit from the client, particularly when the work involved may need a special order of products or resources. Your client may want a full head of coloured hair extensions and this may result in a special order being placed. The cost of this resource must be considered at the time of consultation and a reasonable deposit secured from your client.

LOCATION, LOCATION, LOCATION!

The location of your salon is important. If your salon is situated away from the town centre or in a village this may not attract passing trade. Although you will have to pay more for building rent if situated in the town centre, you should consider whether the extra client base attracted outweighs the additional rent. Overheads must be taken into account, for example, electricity, water, semi-consumable resources such as towels, cotton wool, easi meche and foils.

The pricing structure may well be the responsibility of the salon owner or manager. Treatments are usually costed against the amount of time taken and the cost of the products involved. Chemical treatments such as colouring involve a tremendous amount of technical skill, experience, time taken to consult, apply and process the treatment, leading to the expected professional finished result. Think also about the amount of time you have taken to achieve this wonderful result and, as a professional member of staff, how valuable your time is.

Many professional people charge by the hour and if you think about how much you would like to earn per hour, this will form a basis on how to calculate the likely costs of your client's treatment in your salon.

Everything has a cost attached, so please do remember to add the cost of the consumable and semi-consumable resources together with the cost of the overheads to operate the salon to a professional standard. The cost of the junior answering the telephone down to the cost of buying the coffee, milk and biscuits must all be taken into account.

Location, location, location

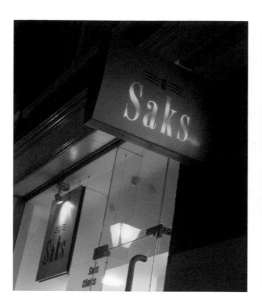

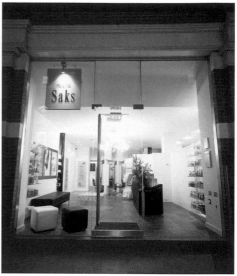

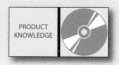
EXCELLENCE POINTS

- It is important to keep in mind and aim to work within the commercial treatment timings of your salon

- The overheads of the salon must be considered to calculate profit and loss for your business

- After-care products should always be recommended to the client

- Make sure you are familiar with the pricing structure and able to communicate it in a professional manner to your client

PROMOTE ADDITIONAL PRODUCTS OR TREATMENTS TO CLIENTS

By promoting additional products to clients, we have the opportunity to increase our income and client base, offering professional advice on using the same products that you retail within the salon.

Ways to promote additional products or treatments to clients include:

- Looking out for opportunities to engage clients in a professional discussion where they can be involved in making an informed decision about the most appropriate product or treatment to use on their hair.

- Creating interesting displays to promote products that are clearly priced. Demonstrate the products to your clients and let them handle them or try them before they buy. Samples to take home are a good idea and offer a professional service without the hard sell.

- Visual displays with relevant printed information will help the client to make an informed decision regarding the suitability of the product.

TIP

Technology is always going through periods of development and products and techniques are changing all the time. Scientists and chemists are constantly striving to bring you, the professional stylist, the best possible product for your clients use, both at home and in the salon, so make sure you keep up to date with new products and trends in the industry.

TIP

Hold seminars in your salon for technical demonstrations and updates of products and techniques. Invite your main colour supplier into your salon to update staff and offer the opportunity for all levels of staff to become more familiar with the treatments and products you as a salon are using. Regular training sessions for all staff will benefit the salon and its business collectively.

Your clients will see the varied range of hairdressing products when they go shopping to the chemist or supermarket. Might they be surprised that their own professional stylist has not recommended a suitable product? They must be aware of what is available from you, the professional. This will encourage them to return to the salon for either a product or treatment or both.

Think about when you would want to discuss the benefits of a product. Common sense would suggest that the best time to discuss *how* to use the product is when you are using it.

Top tips for recommendations

1 Don't sell, recommend. As a hairdresser you have the expertise to advise on the correct hair care for every client

2 Use products at the backwash to prompt the conversation with the client

3 Try it, you might like it – experiment with products so you are confident recommending them to clients

4 Read all about it! – use product sleeves to give on-shelf information about retail and personalise them with your comments

5 Try before you buy – offer mini samples to clients to introduce them to products

6 'Pocket a pound' – for every treatment/retail product sold the stylist receives a pound. A great incentive!

Top tips for merchandising

1 First impressions last – make sure your window is clear, branded and relevant to any salon promotion

2 Shop till you drop – create room in the waiting area for the retail stand to give clients space and time to browse products

3 Don't be afraid of change – if products aren't selling change their position to somewhere more eyecatching and watch sales rise

4 Make it relevant – create displays with a seasonal theme – a Christmas window display or a Summer hair care feature

5 If you have to ask you can't afford it – display prices clearly for clients

TIP ✔

Always offer a future appointment before the client leaves the salon. Your client can then plan ahead and it also allows you to ensure you are meeting your clients needs in terms of an up to date colour and style.

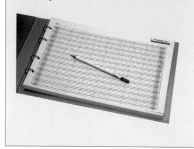

TIP ✔

For those client details stored on a computer, the salon must register with the Data Protection Registrar.

Your client may want to see, touch and possibly smell the product. A little psychology can go a long way when working with clients. Give your clients time to think and ask questions about the product and offer suitable advice on maintaining their hair colour. Too much information at once is sometimes a little too much to deal with.

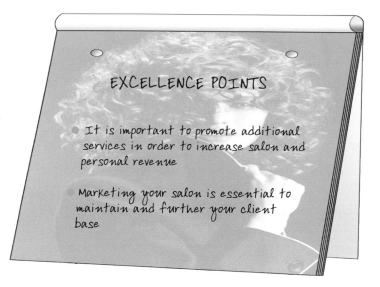

EXCELLENCE POINTS

- It is important to promote additional services in order to increase salon and personal revenue

- Marketing your salon is essential to maintain and further your client base

SALON AND LEGAL REQUIREMENTS

All clients must be asked if they are happy to have their personal and professional details recorded, either on a hand-written record card or entered onto a computer and kept as a professional record. If they wish, clients must have access to their own personal records as and when requested.

Your responsibilities under the Data Protection Act 1998 are to make sure that you:

- obtain and process clients' personal and professional data fairly and lawfully
- hold information only for the purposes specified, such as hairdressing treatments
- disclose this information only to staff who are employed in your salon for professional purposes
- hold information which is adequate for the purpose and which is relevant.

Confidentiality

All clients are entitled to your absolute discretion. Clients have placed themselves in your trust and as a practising professional you must ensure that all manual record cards detailing personal and professional information are stored in a locked cabinet.

Only professional staff must access client records stored on a computer for the sole purpose of the salon's business and must only discuss client information for professional purposes. All client processes should be recorded on a client record card and this procedure must be completed on every visit.

CONSUMER PROTECTION ACT 1987

This act follows European Directives to protect the buyer from unsafe products. The Act is designed to help safeguard the customer from products that do not reach a reasonable level of safety. It would not, therefore, be in your best interests to retail chemical products which could potentially result in harm. The Consumer and Retail Legislation also requires you to reduce the possible risk to customers from any product that may be potentially dangerous.

SOME EMPLOYMENT ISSUES IN THE SALON

Equal opportunities

Your salon will be legally bound to apply the principles of equal opportunities to its staff and clients. Wherever practicable, the salon and its staff must support the principles of equal opportunities whereby unfair discrimination on the basis of race, religion, nationality, ethnic origin, colour, disability, marital status or gender is opposed.

Every possible step needs to be taken to make sure that all individuals are treated equally and fairly. No one must be discriminated against whether they are a member of staff, a client or a visitor to the salon.

Disability Discrimination Act

Employers have a duty to take reasonable steps to prevent placing disabled people who are employees or applicants for employment at a substantial disadvantage in comparison with people who are not disabled.

The following are treated as 'physical features' whether permanent or temporary:

- any feature arising from the design or construction of a building on the premises
- any feature or any approach to, an exit from or access to such a building
- any fixtures, fittings, furnishings, equipment or materials in or on the premises.

A disabled person is a person who has a disability or a long-term health condition that has an impact on their day to day lives and their ability to carry out day to day activities.

It is unlawful for a service provider to discriminate against disabled people, e.g. by refusing to provide them with a service.

As of 1 October 2004 service providers are also required to make physical alterations to buildings when their design or construction makes it impossible or unreasonably difficult for disabled people to gain access to them to use services provided inside.

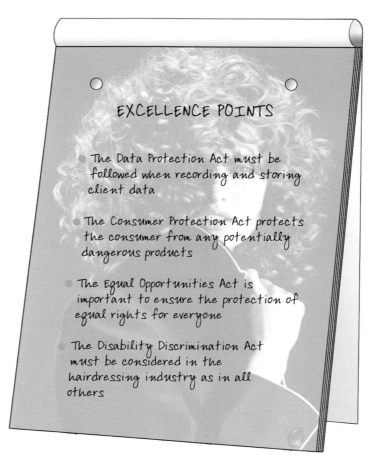

EXCELLENCE POINTS

- The Data Protection Act must be followed when recording and storing client data

- The Consumer Protection Act protects the consumer from any potentially dangerous products

- The Equal Opportunities Act is important to ensure the protection of equal rights for everyone

- The Disability Discrimination Act must be considered in the hairdressing industry as in all others

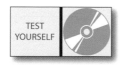

TEST YOURSELF

Testing and essential knowledge

Assessment of knowledge and understanding

Test yourself on the content of this chapter by answering these questions. This will help you to prepare for your Essential knowledge/Written test.

1   Describe effective communication.

2   Give three examples of non-verbal communication.

3   Give three examples of verbal communication.

4   List three topics of conversation that should be avoided in the salon.

5   Why do you need to carry out hair sensitivity and skin allergy tests?

6   What might be present in the hair if you were to take an incompatibility test?

7 Describe pediculous capitis.

8 Differentiate between the features and benefits of a hair style.

9 What does consultation mean?

10 What does analysis mean?

11 What tests are carried out during consultation and why are they important?

12 Copy the table below and complete it.

	Purpose of test	How do you do it?	Expected result	When to do the test	Potential consequences of not carrying out the test
Elasticity test					
Porosity test					
Incompatibility test					
Skin allergy test					
Strand test					

13 Copy the table below and complete it indicating how the results of the listed tests can influence the colouring service.

	Test results	Course of action
Elasticity test	Hair breaks or remains stretched Hair returns to normal	
Porosity test	Hair feels rough Hair feels smooth	
Incompatibility test	No change to hair or liquid Slight increase in temperature of liquid Hair changes colour Liquid bubbles or fizzes	
Skin allergy test	Positive reaction Negative reaction	
Strand test	Hair colour is the required result Hair colour is not required result	

14 Give three reasons why it is important to follow the manufacturer's instructions for skin allergy testing.

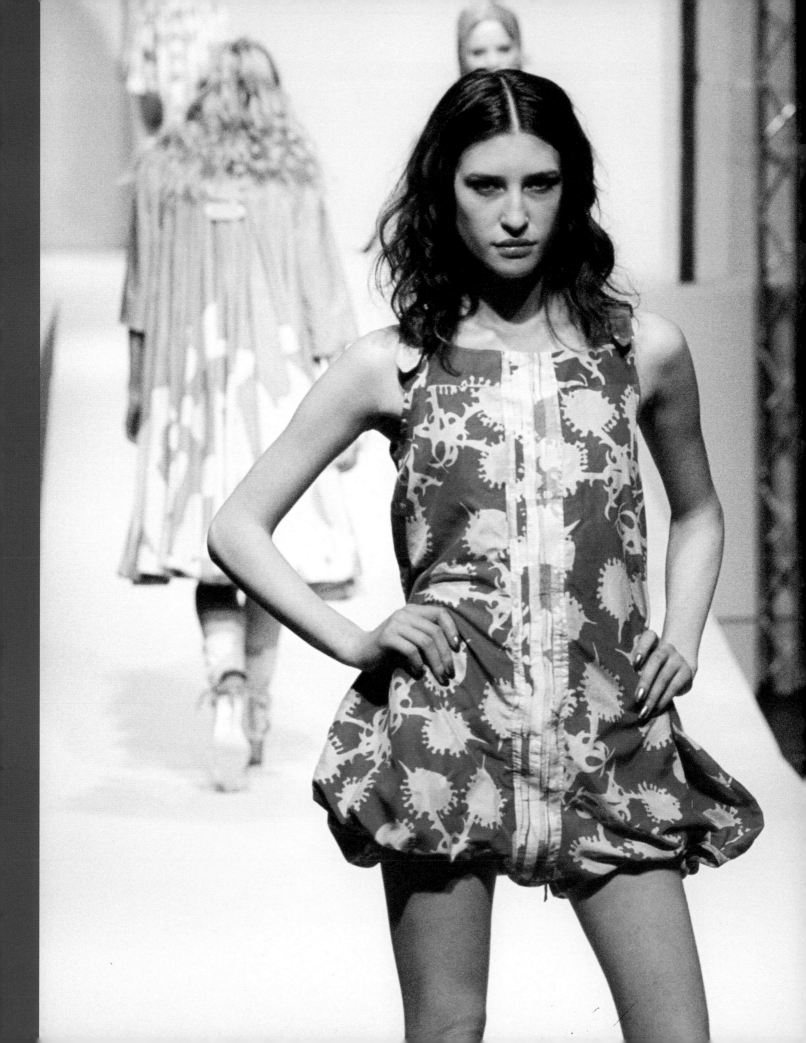

You and Health and Safety in the salon

'Why did you decide to be a colourist?'
'Because I'm really excited by the Health and Safety requirements.'

That's probably not what happened. And if you want to make a fashion statement, you wouldn't choose an apron and disposable gloves. So let's be honest, health and safety is not the most thrilling part of a career, but it is increasingly important. There might have been a time when 'Now Wash Your Hands' was all you needed to know, but things have moved on.

In an industry where you're working with electrical equipment, chemical substances and the public, health and safety is important in three key areas: your employers' responsibilities to you and your colleagues; your responsibility to your colleagues and yourself and your responsibility to your customers.

Attention to health and safety is as much a part of customer service as good communication, and is a sign of your professionalism. At the most basic level, you'd think twice about going back to a dirty and neglected salon, no matter how brilliant the cut and colour.

chapter 6

YOU AND HEALTH AND SAFETY IN THE SALON

Learning objectives

This chapter discusses the health and safety requirements and policies that you will need to know about if you are to work safely and responsibly in the salon: safety and comfort, for both you and your client, are as important as the beauty of hair. In *you and Health and Safety in the salon*, we will consider:

- **The Health and Safety at Work Act (1974)**

- **The Workplace (Health, Safety and Welfare) Regulations (1992)**

- **The Manual Handling Operations Regulations (1992)**

- **The Provision and Use of Work Equipment at Work Regulations (1998)**

- **The Personal Protective Equipment (PPE) at Work Regulations (1992)**

- **The Control of Substances Hazardous to Health Regulations (COSHH) (1999)**

- **The Electricity at Work Regulations (1989)**

- **Reporting of Injuries, Diseases and Dangerous Occurrences Regulations (1995)**

- **Who is responsible for health and safety at work**

- **Making sure you can identify the hazards and risks at work**

- **Enabling you to reduce hazards and risks by operating safe practices at work**

G1 Ensure your actions reduce risks to health & safety

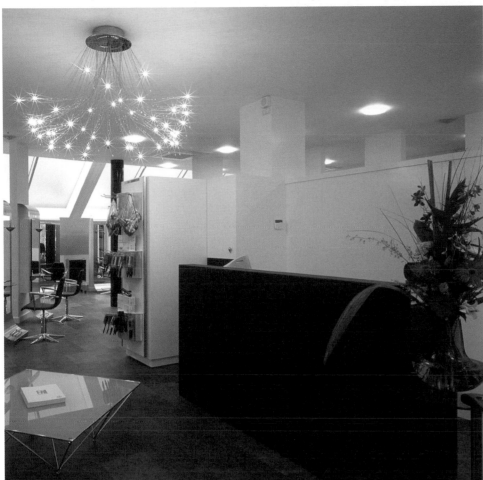

A clean, tidy salon will enhance the salon experience for your client

Saks, Covent Garden

SAFETY AND COMFORT FOR BOTH YOU AND YOUR CLIENT

Whatever work role you have, everyone is required to behave safely and professionally. You must take reasonable care for the health and safety of yourself and others who may be affected by what you do. You must always be responsible for your own behaviour and make sure that your actions do not cause a health and safety risk and you must also co-operate with your employer, owner or manager to ensure that health and safety procedures can be followed.

To work in the hairdressing industry, you will need to demonstrate that you understand the health and safety requirements and policies in the salon. These provide the employer with an approved code of practice for maintaining a safe and secure working environment. You should be constantly improving your own working practices and work areas, preventing any risk of you or others being harmed. This chapter covers the health and safety duties for everyone in the hairdressing industry; it relates directly to the current Habia (Hair and Beauty Industry Authority) occupational standards for hairdressing.

LEGISLATION

The Health and Safety at Work Act (1974)

The Health and Safety at Work Act (1974) covers everyone whether you are an employed person or self-employed, visitors to the salon, including technical representatives, and clients. The Act covers a variety of working practices and is linked to many associated pieces of legislation covering your specific job role. It informs both employer and employee with respect to many aspects of health and safety within the workplace. This act covers most of the relevant legislation that applies to hairdressing and salon employees.

It outlines everybody's duties and responsibilities, including employers, who have slightly different obligations.

The Act's key message is:

It is your duty to maintain the health and safety of yourself and others in the workplace who may be affected by your actions.

The Workplace (Health, Safety and Welfare) Regulations (1992)

This act replaced most of the Office, Shops and Railway Premises Act 1963. It covers a set of benchmarks to cover the legal requirements required in a working environment such as ventilation, indoor temperature, lighting, seating and workstations, windows, doors, gates and walls, staff facilities for eating, rest, drinking water, toilets and room dimensions.

The Act's key message is:

When working in the salon you must maintain a safe and healthy working environment.

The Manual Handling Operations Regulations (1992)

Assess the contents and weight of any box before you attempt to move it, and if need be, empty part of the contents before lifting, or perhaps ask for the help of another member of staff.

You must be shown how to lift heavy objects properly. Always bend your knees and keep your back straight. Think about what you are lifting and where it is going to go. Do you have a safe passageway to carry this load and where are you going to store it? Plan your route and remove any obstructions. It is important that you consider basic health and safety while carrying out day-to-day duties such as unpacking heavy orders of stock.

The Act's key message is:

This act provides guidelines on how to protect yourself, whilst minimising risks to yourself when lifting heavy objects.

Safe lifting practices

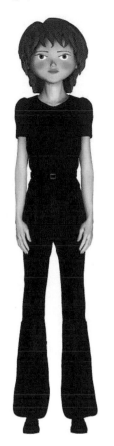

Stand with your feet apart

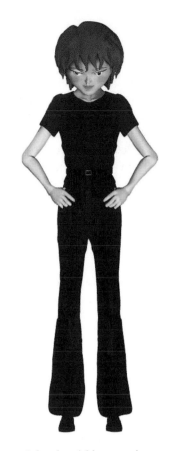

Your weight should be evenly spread over both feet

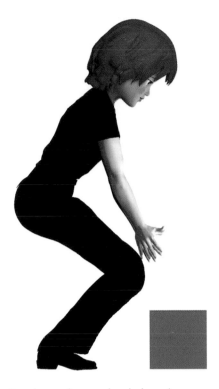

Bend your knees slowly keeping your back straight

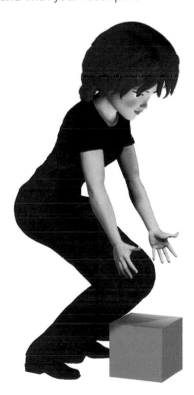

Stand with your feet apart

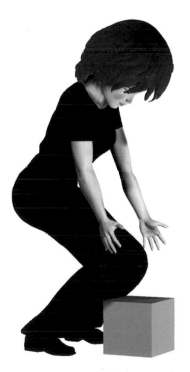

Tuck your chin in towards your chest

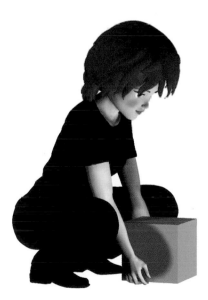

Get a good grip on the base of the box

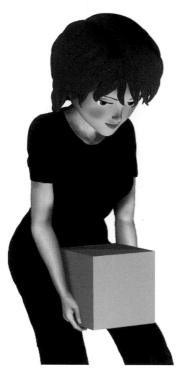

Bring the box to your waist height keeping the lift as smooth as possible

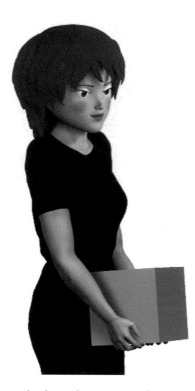

Keep the box close to your body

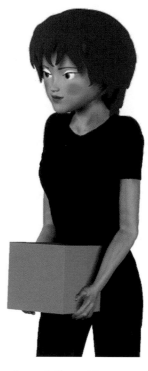

Proceed carefully making sure that you can see where you are going

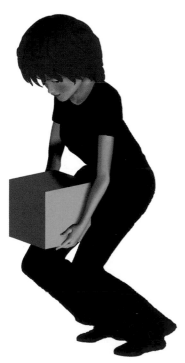

Lower the box, reversing the lifting procedure

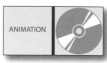

ANIMATION

Safe lifting practices

EXCELLENCE POINTS

● Under the Health and Safety at Work Act (1974) you must maintain reasonable care of yourself and others at work

● The Workplace Regulations state that your employer must maintain a safe and healthy salon for you to work in and where clients can relax in safety while having their hair done

● The Manual Handling Regulations state that you must always take care when you are lifting heavy objects

The Provision and Use of Work Equipment at Work Regulations (1998)

This states the duties for employers and the self-employed when providing work equipment. These regulations also cover the selection of suitable equipment, maintenance, manufacturer information, instruction and training. Specific regulations address the dangers that could arise from operation of the equipment and potential risk of injury.

The Act's key message is:

You must be competent when using tools and equipment in the salon.

The Personal Protective Equipment (PPE) at Work Regulations (1992)

The Personal Protective Equipment (PPE) legislation states that you must wear suitable protective gloves and an apron when dealing with any chemical or harmful substance linked with colouring. You must always wear PPE when using colouring products and clients must be suitably protected during the colour treatment. By ensuring your use of personal protective equipment, you will meet the health and safety regulations and workplace policies. Remember that PPE includes preparing your clients' hair and protecting their skin where necessary prior to any colouring treatment.

The Act's key message is:

Your employer must provide appropriate personal protective equipment when working with chemical treatments and you must always use it when applicable.

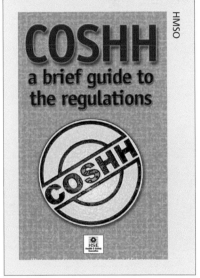

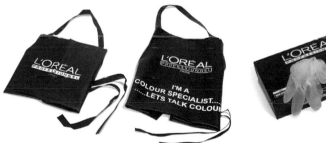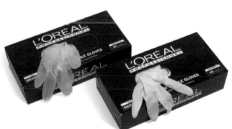

Your employer must provide appropriate personal protective equipment for when you are working in the salon

The Control of Substances Hazardous to Health (COSHH) Regulations (1999)

COSHH is a workplace policy that is relevant to your everyday working practices. Chemicals that are toxic or inflammable such as bleach (pre-lightener), colour, perm lotions, neutralisers and hydrogen peroxide are hazardous and present a high risk. They must be stored, handled, used and disposed of correctly in accordance with COSHH 1993.

ACTIVITY

Make a note of your responsibilities under COSHH in relation to using colouring and bleaching (pre-lightening) products

When using bleach powder consider buying a dust-free product; this will lessen the dangers associated with the inhalation of powder bleach. Ensure that you know how to use all chemicals safely and take safe, professional precautions when using hazardous substances. All colouring products, materials and equipment must be used in accordance with the manufacturer's instructions, salon policy and local by-laws.

This law also applies to retail products. All manufacturers will by law inform you, the professional hairdresser, of all ingredients of each hairdressing product stored in your salon. Many products such as hair spray, mousse, perm lotion and hydrogen peroxide are potentially hazardous and should be stored in a cool, dark, locked, fireproof cabinet, preferably on a low shelf.

The Act's key message is:

Any substances in use in your salon that may be hazardous to health should be stored, handled, used and disposed of according to legislation, manufacturers' instructions and local byelaws.

EXCELLENCE POINTS

- The Provision of Work Equipment Act states that employers and the self-employed must provide training in the use of suitable equipment and that it is also maintained to ensure that employees use tools and equipment correctly and safely

- The Personal Protective Equipment Act states that your employer must provide suitable disposable gloves, aprons, gowns and capes when carrying out any chemical process

- The Control of Substances Hazardous to Health Regulations say that you must store, handle, use and dispose of all chemical substances according to local by-laws and manufacturers' instructions

The Electricity at Work Regulations (1989)

The Electricity at Work Regulations 1989 are particularly important, as we often rely heavily on the use of electrical equipment in the hairdressing salon. We need to be careful prior to using pieces of equipment in order that we minimise the risk of accidents to both our clients and ourselves. The salon owner has the responsibility to ensure that a qualified electrician maintains all electrical equipment on a regular basis. Hairdryers, climazons, steamers and roller balls are but a few of the items of electrical equipment linked to colouring and must be Portable Applicance Test (PAT) tested to ensure that all electrical equipment is safe to use on clients.

Your responsibilities under the Electricity at Work Regulations include checking electrical equipment that is used to facilitate the colouring and lightening process. Should any piece of equipment become faulty you must report it, label it faulty and remove it to a safe place where that piece of equipment can be mended. A written record of these tests must be kept and shown to the Health and Safety inspectors if requested.

The Act's key message is:

All electrical equipment must be used appropriately with precaution, checked and tested, the position of plugs and sockets must be safe and the space you are working in must have adequate lighting. Any faulty and damaged equipment must be removed from use, labelled and reported to a responsible person.

The salon's policy for handling and storing electrical equipment is that we:

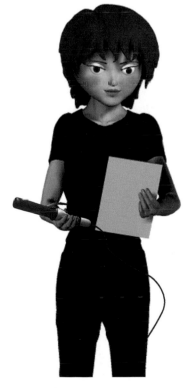

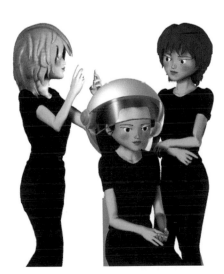

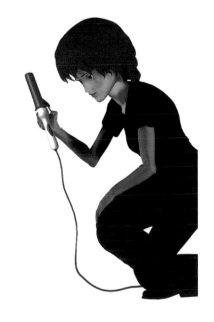

- Know how to use it
- Be trained in its use
- Use it only for the purpose intended

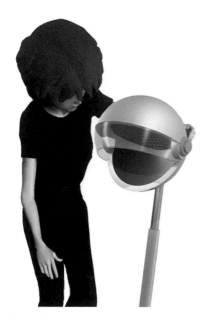

• Visually check prior to use

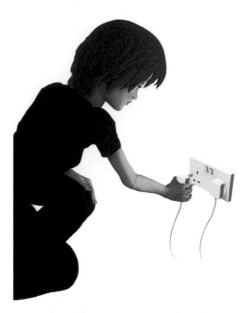

• Isolate the power supply when finished

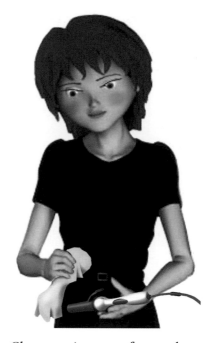

• Clean equipment after each use

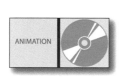

Electrical equipment

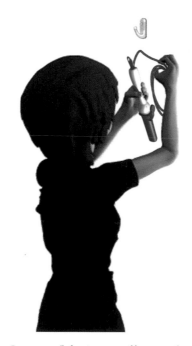

• Store safely, in an allocated area

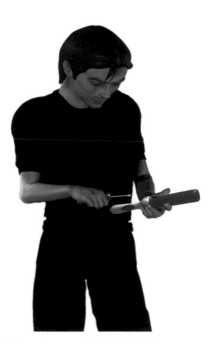

• Have it tested regularly by a qualified electrician.

Reporting of Injuries, Diseases and Dangerous Occurrences Regulations (RIDDOR) (1995)

All injuries must be reported to the member of staff responsible for health and safety. This includes injuries involving clients, visitors and staff. The salon accident book must be completed with basic personal details of the person or persons involved together with a detailed description of the incident, and this must be reported to the salon owner. There may be legal consequences because of the injury and all witnesses must provide a clear and accurate account of what took place.

The Act's key message is:

You must report:

- Any fatal accidents
- Any major injury sustained while at work
- Work-related diseases
- Any potentially dangerous event that takes place at work
- Accidents causing more than three days absence from work.

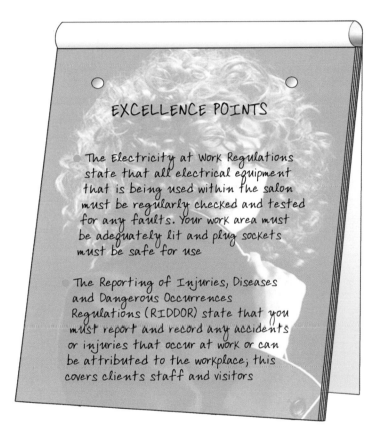

EXCELLENCE POINTS

The Electricity at Work Regulations state that all electrical equipment that is being used within the salon must be regularly checked and tested for any faults. Your work area must be adequately lit and plug sockets must be safe for use

The Reporting of Injuries, Diseases and Dangerous Occurrences Regulations (RIDDOR) state that you must report and record any accidents or injuries that occur at work or can be attributed to the workplace; this covers clients staff and visitors

HAZARDS AND RISKS

Although the salon is a great place to work in, there are some risks or hazardous areas. The Health and Safety Act covers all full or part-time employees and unpaid workers (such as work placement assistants). You will need to be aware of your legal duties for health and safety in the workplace as required by the Health and Safety at Work Act 1974.

The Health and Safety Executive is the body appointed to support and enforce health and safety in the workplace. They have defined the two concepts of hazard and risk:

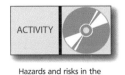

ACTIVITY

Hazards and risks in the salon

Hazard symbols

- A hazard – something with the potential to cause harm
- A risk – the likelihood of the hazard's potential being realised.

Hazards

A hazard has the potential to cause harm and you must identify working practices within the salon which could harm yourself or other people. All staff are required to make sure that the salon equipment and the workplace are well-maintained and safe to use.

For example:

- A light bulb that needs replacing is a hazard. If it is just one out of several it presents very little risk, but if it is the only light on a stairwell, it is a very high risk.
- A bowl of tint or bleach on a trolley top is a potential hazard that can fall off, causing spillage on clothes, creating a slippery surface on the floor unless cleared away immediately.

> **TIP**
>
> Although parents and guardians are primarily responsible for their child's care while in the salon, salon staff are required to keep all hazardous substances out of harm's way.

> **TIP**
>
> In environments such as hairdressing salons, warm moist atmospheres are perfect breeding grounds, therefore it is essential to keep the salon well ventilated to reduce the risk of cross-infection.

> **TIP**
>
> Good ventilation is important when mixing colours and bleaches and when using colouring preparations. Windows and/or an air vent must be opened, as chemicals can be dangerous if inhaled.

Risks

A risk presents the possibility of a hazard causing harm. It is important to remain alert to the presence of hazards in the workplace and it is essential to deal with them properly to make sure that they do not present a risk to yourself, your colleagues or your clients. You must deal with both hazards and risks in accordance with workplace policy and legal requirements.

For example:

- Slippery surfaces are a hazard and must be mopped up promptly, so that you or your client do not risk a slip or a fall.
- A plugged-in hairdryer has been left on a trolley whilst not in use and is a hazard because the trailing cable presents a risk, as someone could trip over the wire.
- Hot water can be hazardous because of the risk of spillages scalding clients.

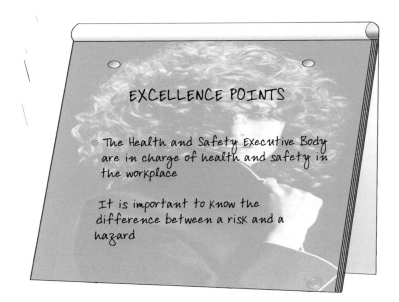

EXCELLENCE POINTS

The Health and Safety Executive Body are in charge of health and safety in the workplace

It is important to know the difference between a risk and a hazard

ACTIVITY

Evidence is important when creating your portfolio and within your own work role. Provide some examples of how you have taken steps to reduce those health and safety risks which you may come into contact within the salon.

RISK ASSESSMENT

Your employer must carry out a risk assessment of all the substances you will use within your work role to determine:

- What the hazards are and in what form, e.g. fluids or gas
- Who will be affected
- How much exposure they will have
- The workplace location, e.g. main salon or stock rooms
- The control measures to minimise the risk
- How these will be monitored
- How much instruction, information and training is required for employees.

You will need to know your salon's workplace policy relating to controlling risks to health and safety and you must be able to identify and evaluate those working practices that are potentially harmful.

The potentially harmful aspects of the workplace are those with the highest risk to you and other people. From the risks arising from any hazards you have identified, you must know which risks you can deal with safely, within the limits of your own job role and authority, and which risks must be reported to a more senior member of staff who is responsible for health and safety in the workplace.

Responsible person

Health and safety regulations state that there must be a responsible person in the salon who will keep all records and be the main contact for all the staff in the salon. That person would need to contact the Health and Safety Executive if accidents that need reporting occur.

ACTIVITY

Create a family tree of people in your salon, start at the top with the salon owner and work down from that. Indicate each person's name, job title and his or her responsibilities and identify the person that is responsible for reporting any accidents to the Health and Safety Executive.

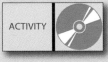

ACTIVITY

Create a family tree

RISKS IN THE SALON

Think about how you position your client to meet the needs of the treatment without causing discomfort. Ensure your own posture and position when you are working minimises fatigue and the risk of injury. This can affect the desired outcome in terms of your client's hairdressing treatment. Keep your work area clean and tidy during the treatment, positioning your tools and equipment for ease of use. This will minimise the risk of cross-infection or infestation, leaving all surfaces hygienically clean.

Get into the habit of using working methods that:

- Minimise the wastage of products. Only mix products that you want to use at any one time. Weighing products will give a more accurate amount each time.

- Minimise the risk of cross-infection by using clean tools and equipment. Your clients are entitled to clean tools and equipment – always.

- Make constructive use of your time. This will help save your valuable time during the day and make effective use of your client's time and that of salon staff.

- Minimise the risk of harm or injury to yourself and others that may be affected by your actions. Take care when using hazardous products such as bleach (pre-lighteners), decolourants, hydrogen peroxide and colouring products.

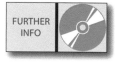

FURTHER INFO

Good posture

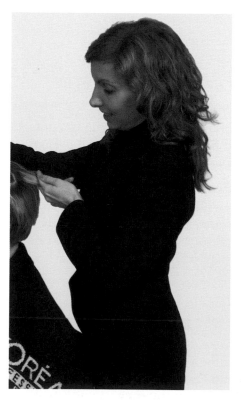

Good posture – standing

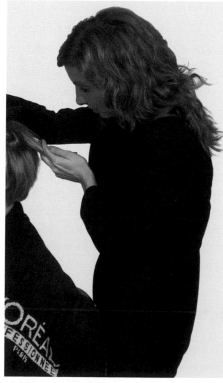

Bad posture

Positioning your tools for efficient working practices

By positioning your tools within easy reach, you will make constructive use of your time as well as present a professional image to your clients, therefore reducing the overall time that your client is in the salon. Remove waste immediately at the end of all colouring and lightening treatments and dispose of in accordance with local bylaws. This will ensure that all waste is removed correctly leaving your working surfaces free from any risk or hazard.

Personal conduct policy

Salon policy for personal conduct should cover:

- General behaviour in the salon
- Whether or not smoking is allowed
- Where eating and drinking can take place
- Whether use of prohibited drugs would lead to disciplinary action
- How to use equipment correctly
- The systems that are in place with reference to timekeeping
- How staff absence should be reported
- How to inform the salon of any illness that will involve time away from work
- The dress code of the salon.

TIP

Never climb onto furniture, shelves or boxes – always use a ladder and get a colleague to hold it steady for you.

ACTIVITY

Produce your own workplace policy including all the above points.

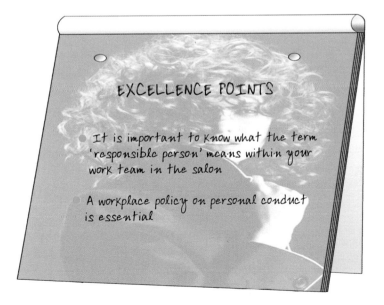

EXCELLENCE POINTS

It is important to know what the term 'responsible person' means within your work team in the salon

A workplace policy on personal conduct is essential

STERILISING YOUR EQUIPMENT

You must use tools and equipment that are clean, safe and fit for their purpose; i.e. tools and equipment identified at the time of consultation must be readily available to use for professional purposes. This means pintail

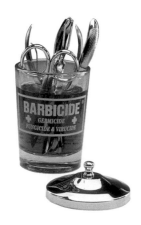

Barbicide

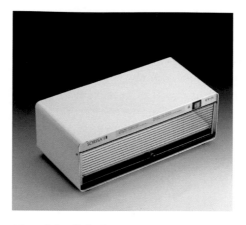

Ultraviolet light box

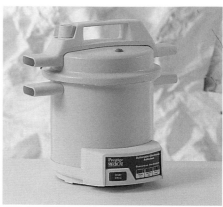

An autoclave

combs to weave sections of hair, highlighting hooks to pull strands of hair through a highlighting cap, professional foil strips to assist colouring etc.

Sterilising equipment

The methods of sterilisation available in salons may include:

- Barbicide
- An ultraviolet light box
- An autoclave.

The most common method of sterilising is barbicide which is quick and easy to use. Barbicide will only inhibit the growth of bacteria and you must read and follow the manufacturer's instructions when making up the solution; you will also need to change it daily.

The ultraviolet light box will prevent the growth of bacteria on tools that are clean and dry: remember to turn your tools over every 15 minutes to keep both sides hygienically clean.

The most successful method of sterilising is the autoclave, which will destroy all living bacteria from the surface of your tools. The importance of sterilising your tools is paramount for a hygienic working environment that will promote a standard of cleanliness to your clients and staff, preventing the risk of cross-infection and infestation.

FIRE

Fire can only occur when three factors are present:

- Fuel
- Air
- Heat.

Should one of these factors be absent or removed, combustion cannot take place. Therefore, it is essential that:

- No heaters are stored next to flammable material, e.g. hydrogen peroxide

- Inflammable stock is stored in a fire proof cabinet
- Aerosols are kept away from any direct heat source including sun light
- There is no smoking in the salon.

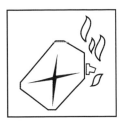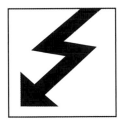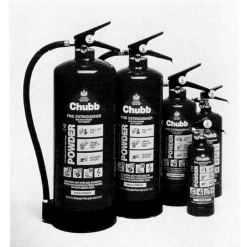

Fire extinguisher symbols   Fire extinguishers

ACTIVITY

Emergency procedures
Draw a plan of your salon indicating:

- The exits for evacuation
- Where the assembly points are
- The location of the fire fighting equipment
- The location of the first aid kit and accident book.

EXCELLENCE POINTS

- There are three methods of sterilisation

- Know how a fire can start and how to take reasonable steps to avoid any incidents of this nature occurring

An example of best practice for
the use of professional products
and techniques from
L'Oréal Professionnel

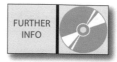

FURTHER
INFO

Best practice

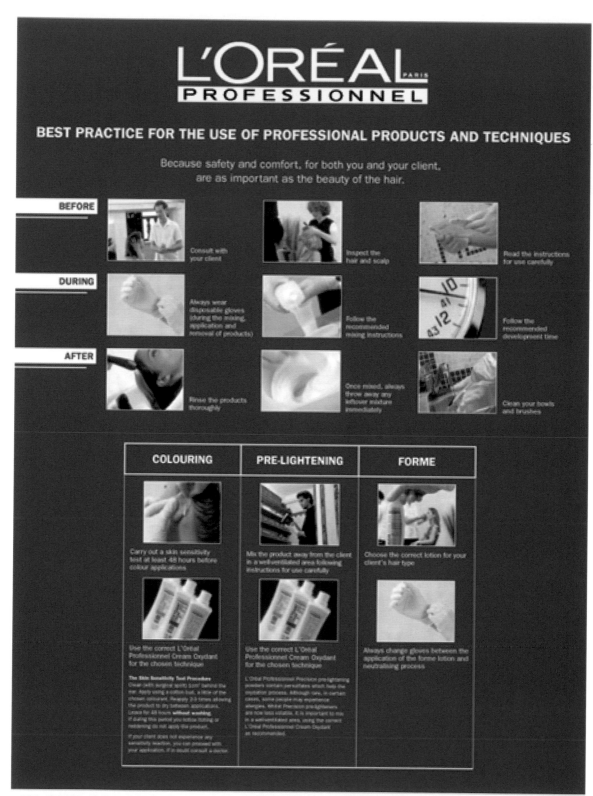

IN THE SALONS OF THE WORLD'S GREATEST HAIRDRESSERS

Assessment of knowledge and understanding

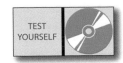

Test yourself on the content of this chapter by answering these questions. This will help you to prepare for your Essential knowledge/Written test.

1 What does the word risk mean?

2 What does the word hazard mean?

3 Give three examples of a hazard that could be found in the salon.

4 What does COSHH mean?

5 Describe your responsibilities as an employee for health and safety in the salon.

6 Who is the person responsible for reporting health and safety matters in the salon?

7 What responsibilities do you have under the Electricity at Work Regulations?

8 What does RIDDOR stand for?

9 Why is it important to deal promptly with health and safety matters?

10 How would you deal with the following:
   (a) Faulty electrical equipment
   (b) Slippery surfaces?

11 Why should you remain alert to the presence of hazards?

12 What could happen if there are obstructions to the entry and exit doors of your salon?

13 Think of three safe practices when using both colouring and bleaching products.

14 What effect may unprofessional behaviour have on your colleagues and clients?

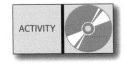

ACTIVITY

Wordsearch

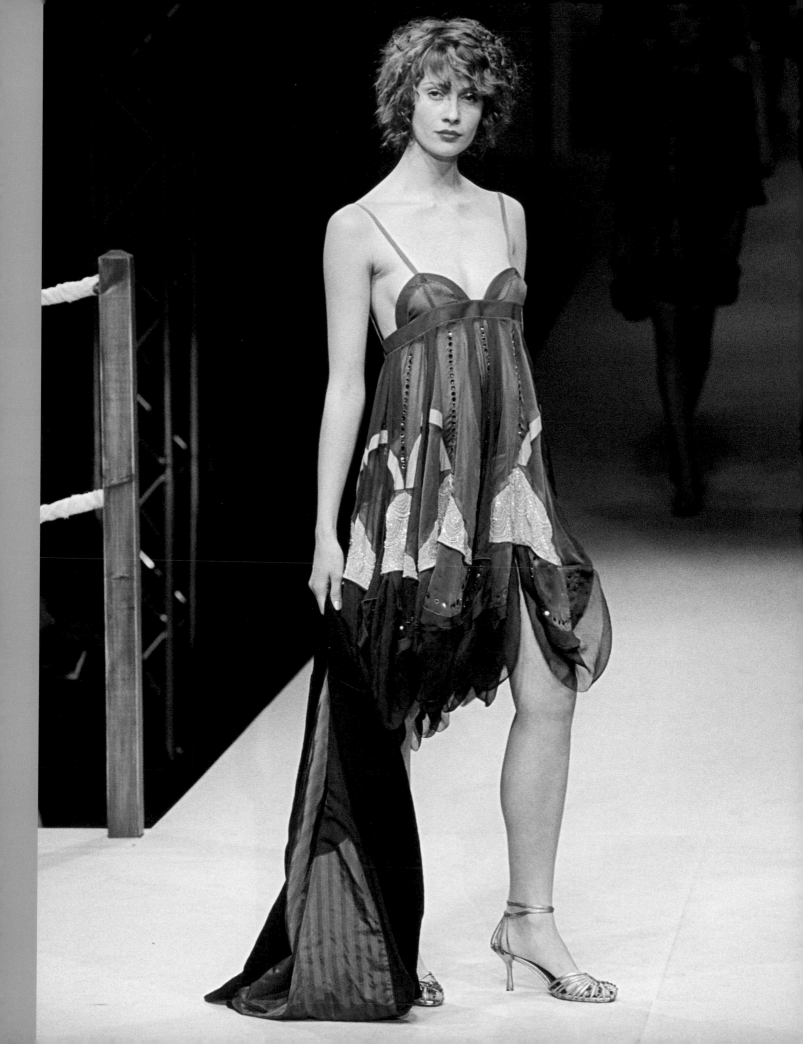

Technique matters

'Our hair is our most visible asset, and the way to make the most of it is to have it professionally coloured.'

Arthur Ehoff, L'Oréal UK

Colour is fun, fashion and image. So what's missing from the list? Colour is money. We've all been to salons where a few sad, dusty colour charts are the only sign of a colour service. Which is very effective ... at turning anyone off the idea. Sometimes a poodle parlour seems a better choice.

About ten per cent of women have their hair coloured, which means that 90 per cent don't. As the average colour bill is higher than a cut and blow dry bill, that's a great opportunity.

According to Robert Soutar at L'Oréal UK, 'in theory, a salon can increase its revenue by 50, 75 or even 100 per cent if it gets the colour business right'. So what's the best way to do it? The first thing is that the colourist is trained to the highest level. But no matter how brilliant you are people need to know about you. Colour postcards, flyers and showcards are effective marketing tools. Existing colour clients can be your best advert, so give them *Introduce a Friend to Colour* cards. Encourage visitors to have their cut coloured, and their colour cut.

Remember that everyone wants to look great. As a colourist, you're one of the best people to make it happen.

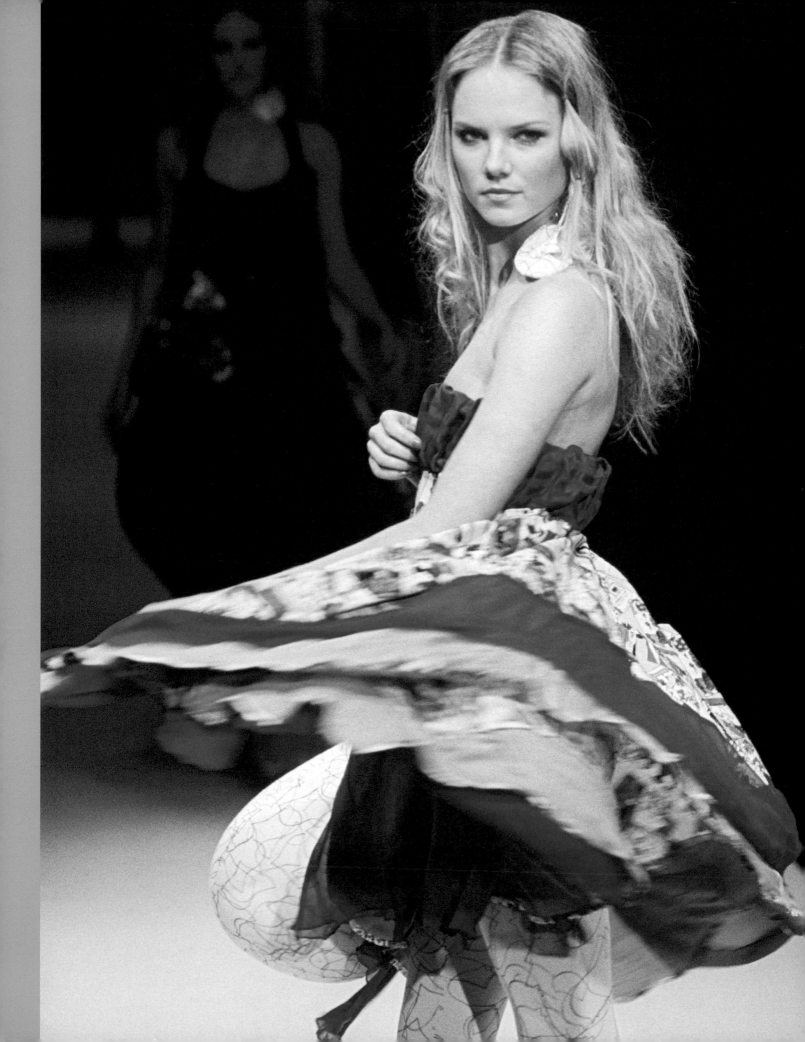

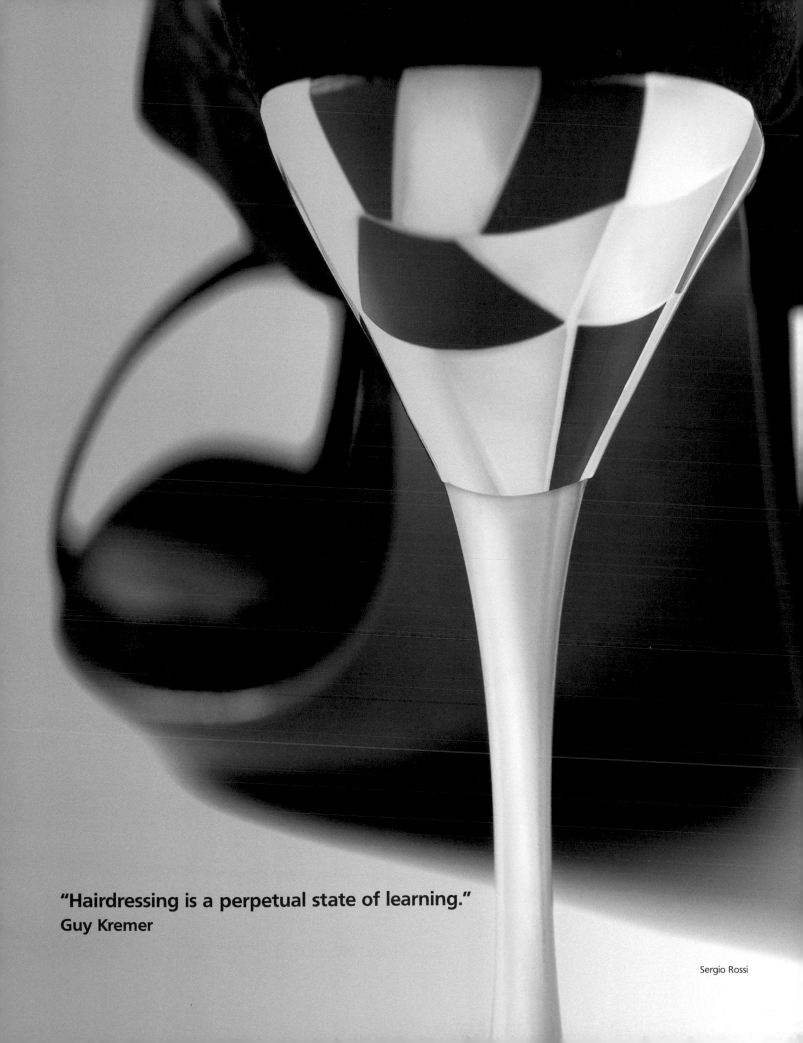

"Hairdressing is a perpetual state of learning."
Guy Kremer

Sergio Rossi

STEPPED

This technique gives a twist to full head highlights and is ideal for long hair.

Step 1

Divide the hair into ten sections.

Step 2

Make two sections at the nape, three sections above the occipital bone, two at the crown and finally three across the top of the head.

Step 3

Working through the back, use alternating lightening and colouring products in sections of fine weaves and slices.

Step 4

On a diagonal angle, take sections across the top of the head from ear to ear and across the forehead, continuing to alternate products.

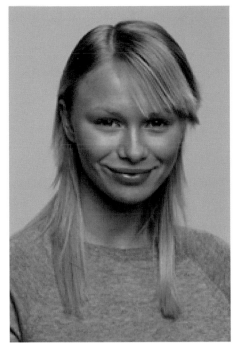

Before colour application

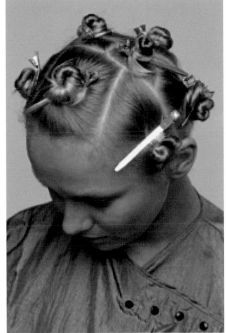

Step 1

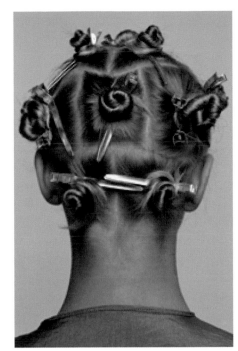

Step 2

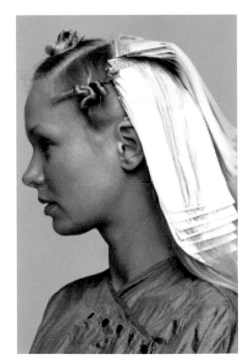

Step 3

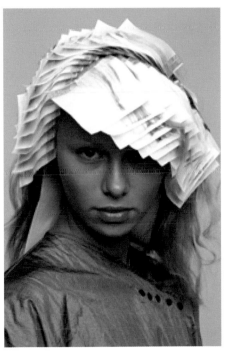

Step 4

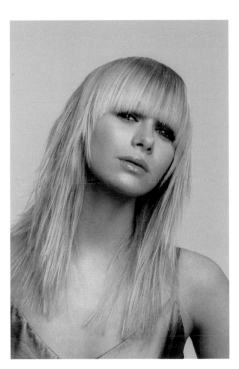

Final colour result

FOCAL PIVOT

This focal pivot is suitable for all lengths of hair with texture and movement.

Step 1

Take two diagonal partings from the crown to the front recession area to form a large triangle on the top of the head and secure.

Step 2

Colour the remaining hair with chosen shade from roots through to lengths and ends.

Step 3

Isolate the hair already coloured using foils or Easi Meche. Take a large slice section and apply a contrasting colour.

Step 4

Continue to work in back to back slices, alternating the contrasting colour with the initial chosen shade.

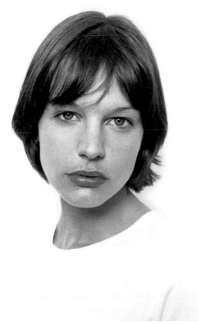

Before colour application

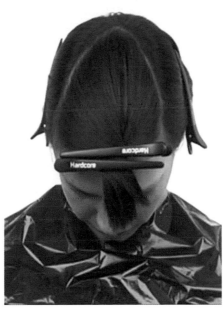

Step 1

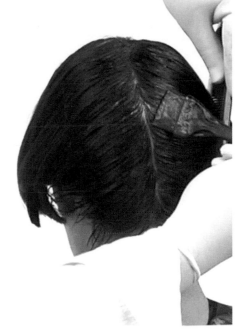

Step 2

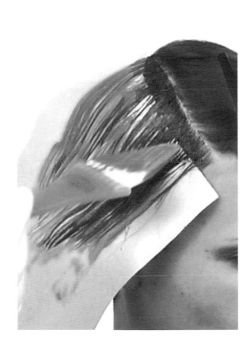

Step 3

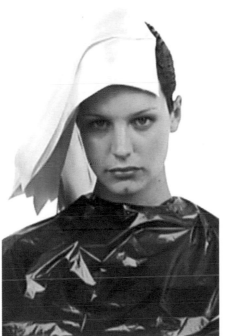

Step 4

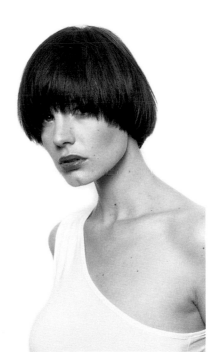

Final colour result

Toni and Guy International Technical Team

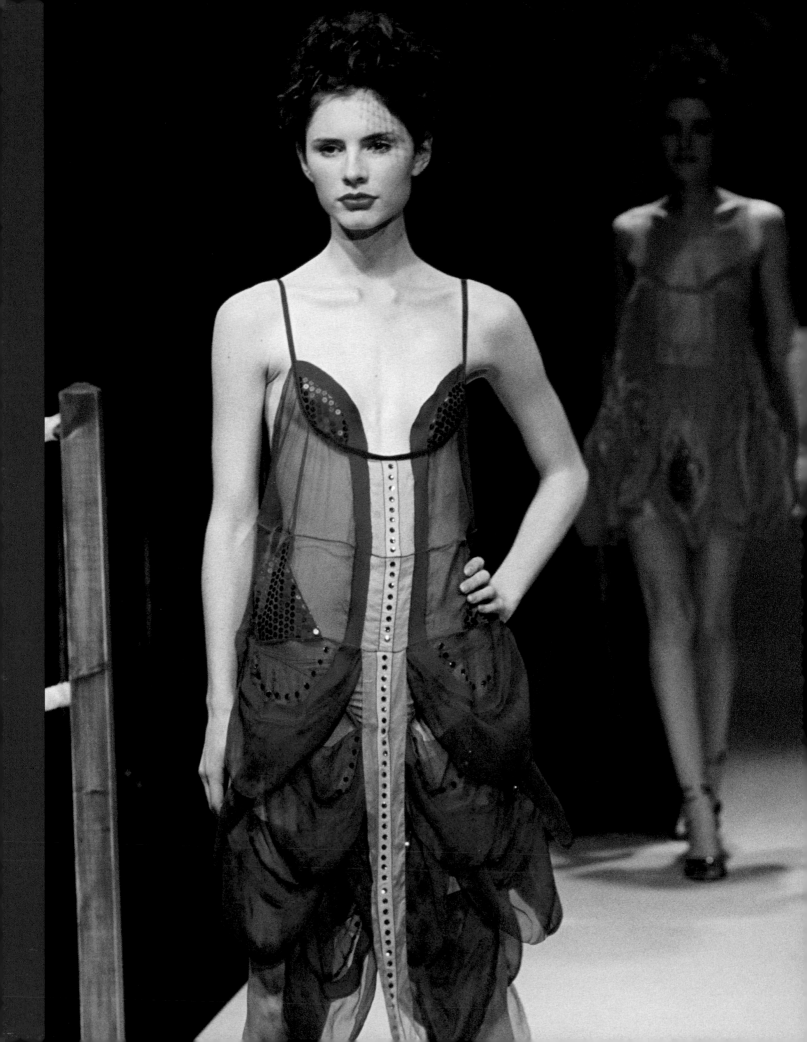

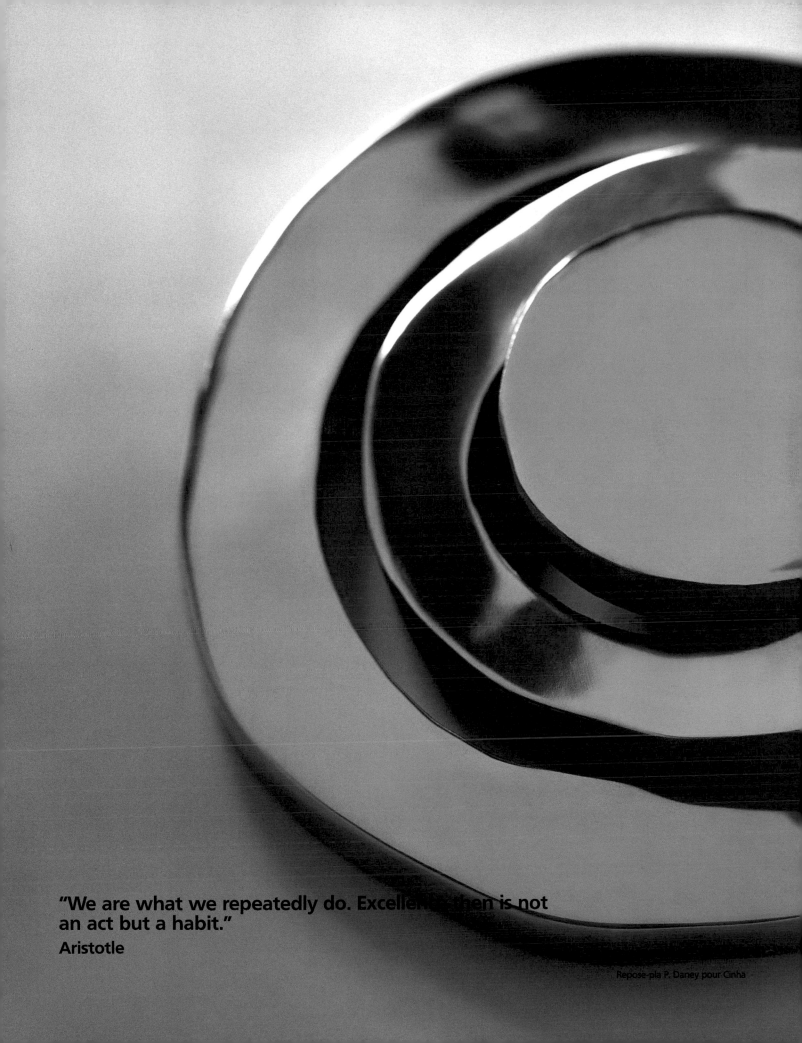

"We are what we repeatedly do. Excellence, then is not an act but a habit."
Aristotle

Repose-pla P. Daney pour Cinha

CASHMERE BLONDE

This technique makes natural, baby-blonde hair as soft and luxurious as cashmere, and will never go out of fashion.

Step 1

Analyse client's hair and scalp prior to bleach (pre-lightener) application to check for cuts and abrasions.

Step 2

Apply product to the root area taking care not to overlap to lengths and ends.

Step 3

Monitor until the degree of lift has been achieved, always develop in accordance with instructions.

Step 4

Apply toner quickly and evenly throughout the hair.

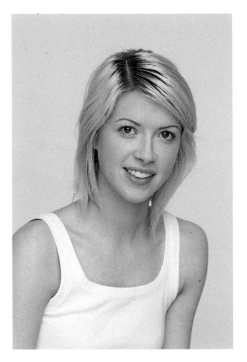

Before colour application

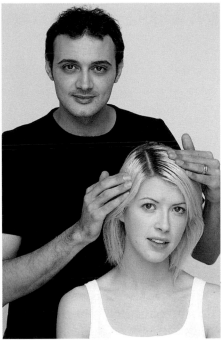

Step 1

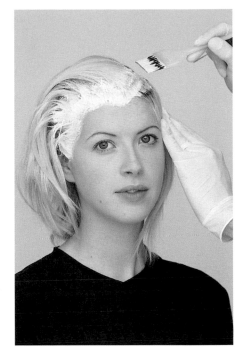

Step 2

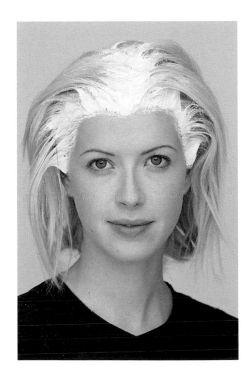

Step 3

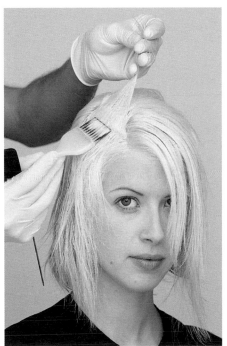

Step 4

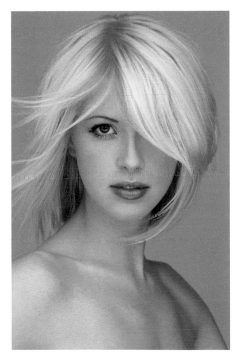

Final colour result

Hair by Trevor Sorbie Art Team in association with L'Oréal Professionnel.
Creative Director Angelo Seminara, Technical Director Nathan Walker

REVERSED DIAGONAL HORSESHOE

A reversed diagonal horseshoe technique is suitable for all lengths of hair.

Step 1

Make a horseshoe section on the top and then sub divide into three parts.

Step 2

Work diagonally through the section taking slices and isolating in foils or Easi Meche.

Step 3

Begin the second section by taking diagonal sections again but working in the opposite direction to the first section.

Step 4

The final section is then worked parallel to the first one but opposite to the second section.

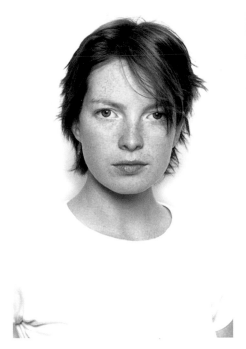

Before colour application

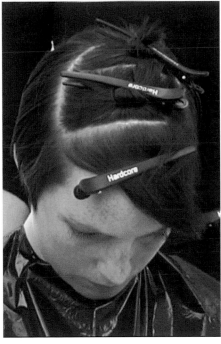

Step 1

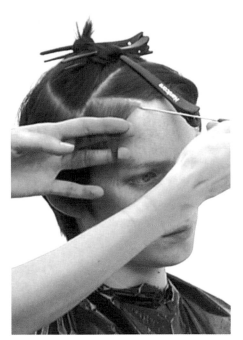

Step 2

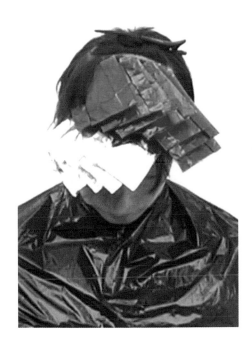

Step 3

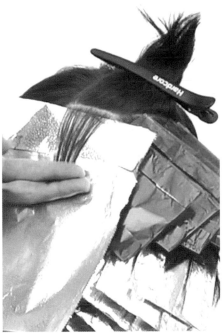

Step 4

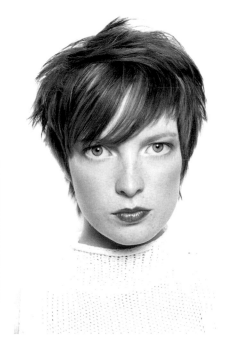

Final colour result

Toni & Guy International Technical Team

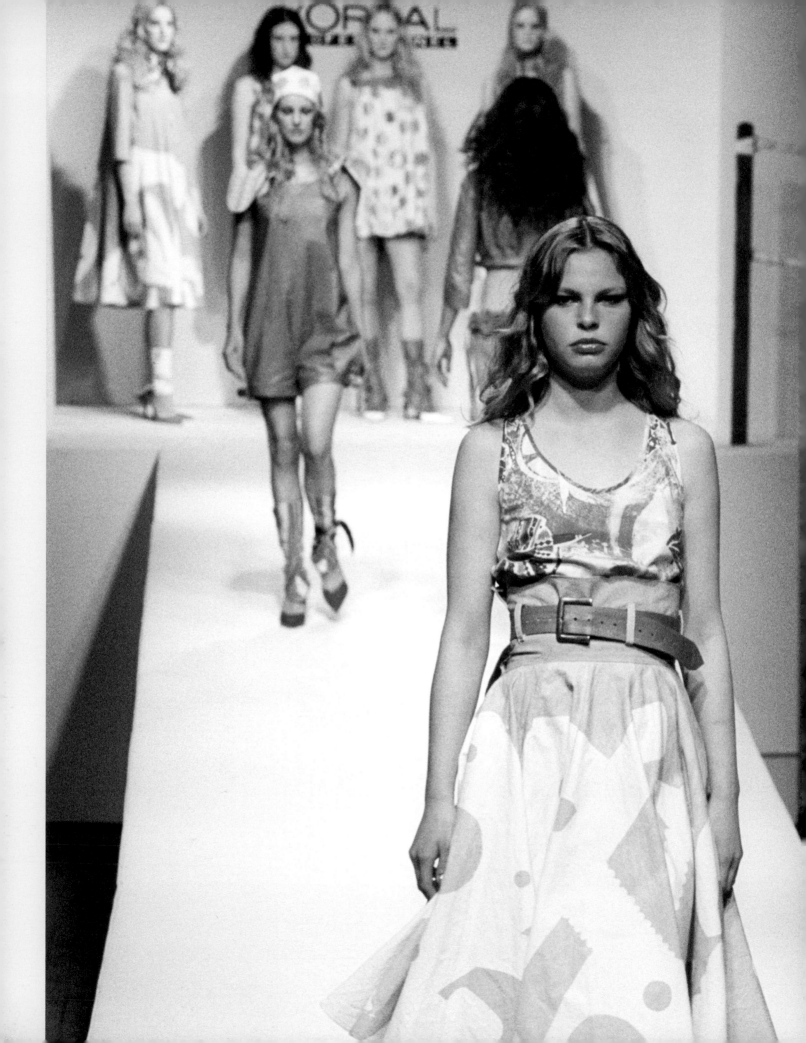

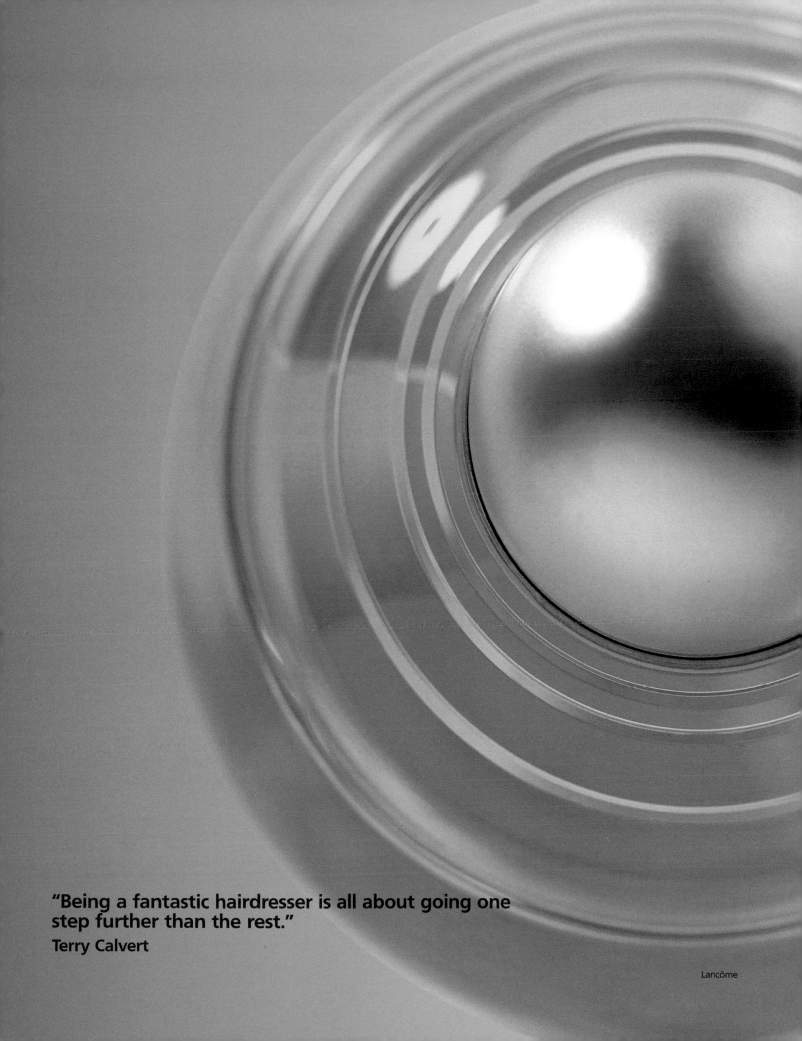

"Being a fantastic hairdresser is all about going one step further than the rest."
Terry Calvert

Lancôme

SWIRL

This technique creates a natural, sun-kissed effect for both men and women.

Step 1

Create a circular section at the top, slightly off centre.

Step 2

Take a halo section underneath the circle, working from the parting to the opposite ear progressively.

Step 3

Make diagonal slices through this section and apply a lightening product through the lengths and ends of each slice, isolate with foils or Easi Meche.

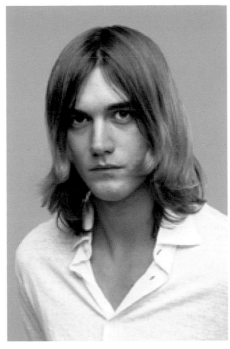

Before colour application

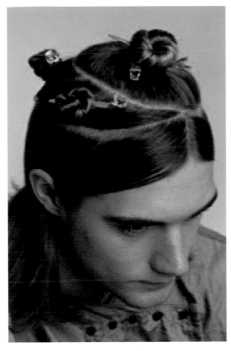

Step 1

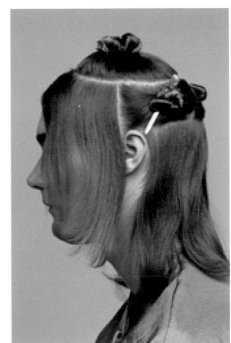

Step 2

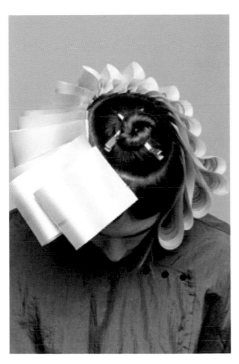

Step 3

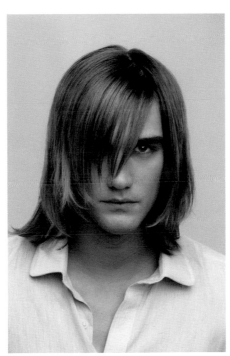

Final colour result

ALTERNATIVE T-SECTION

The alternative T-section is suitable for long layers and one-length shapes.

Step 1

A triangular section is taken from the front recession area on both sides to the top crown.

Step 2

The triangle is then sub-divided in to two parts from the centre of one of the sides to the centre of the front hairline.

Step 3

On the smallest section work through diagonally with large weaves, isolating the hair with foils or Easi Meche until you reach the top of the section.

Step 4

The opposite larger section is worked by taking slices on a slight diagonal.

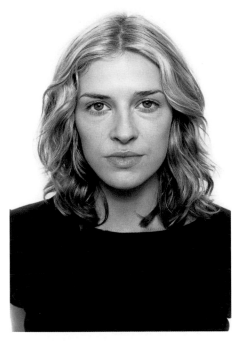

Before colour application

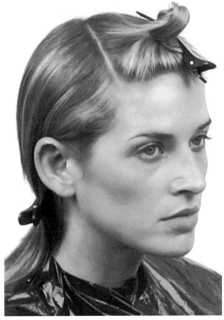

Step 1

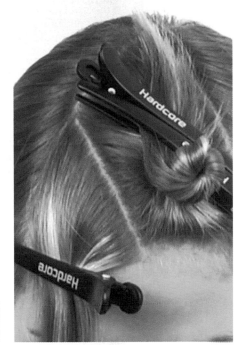

Step 2

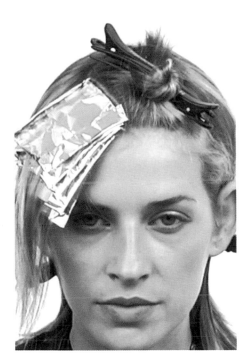

Step 3

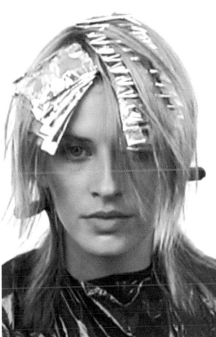

Step 4

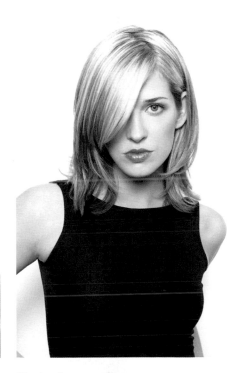

Final colour result

Toni & Guy International Technical Team

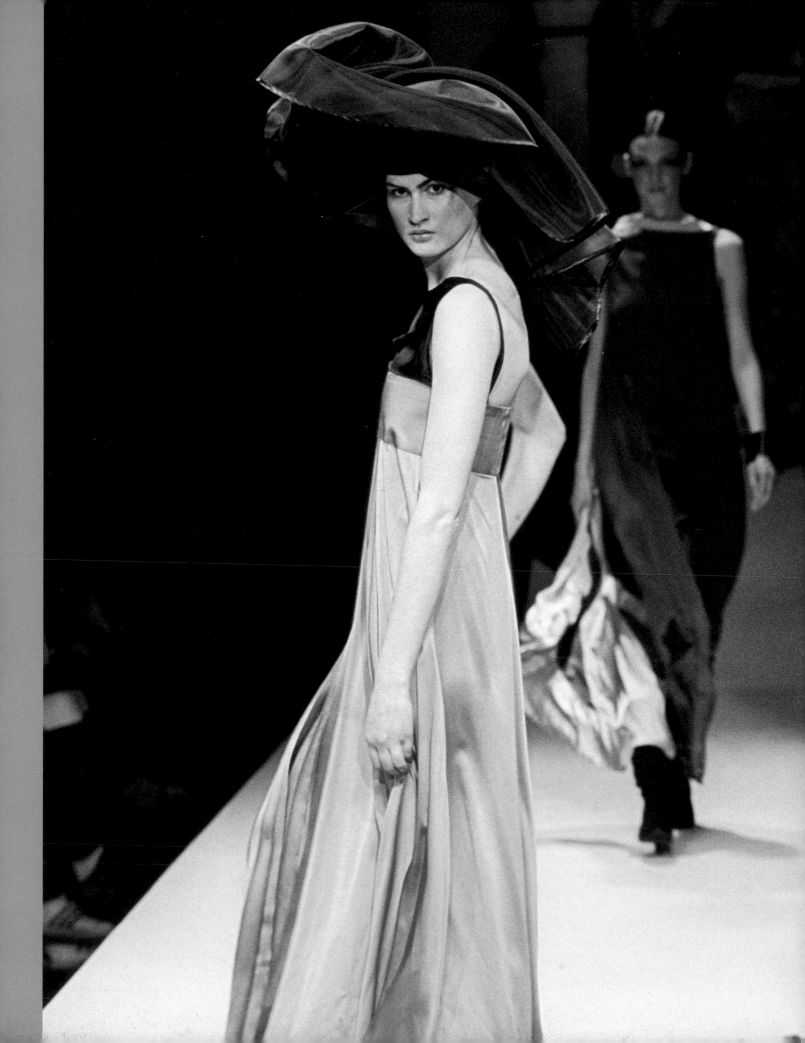

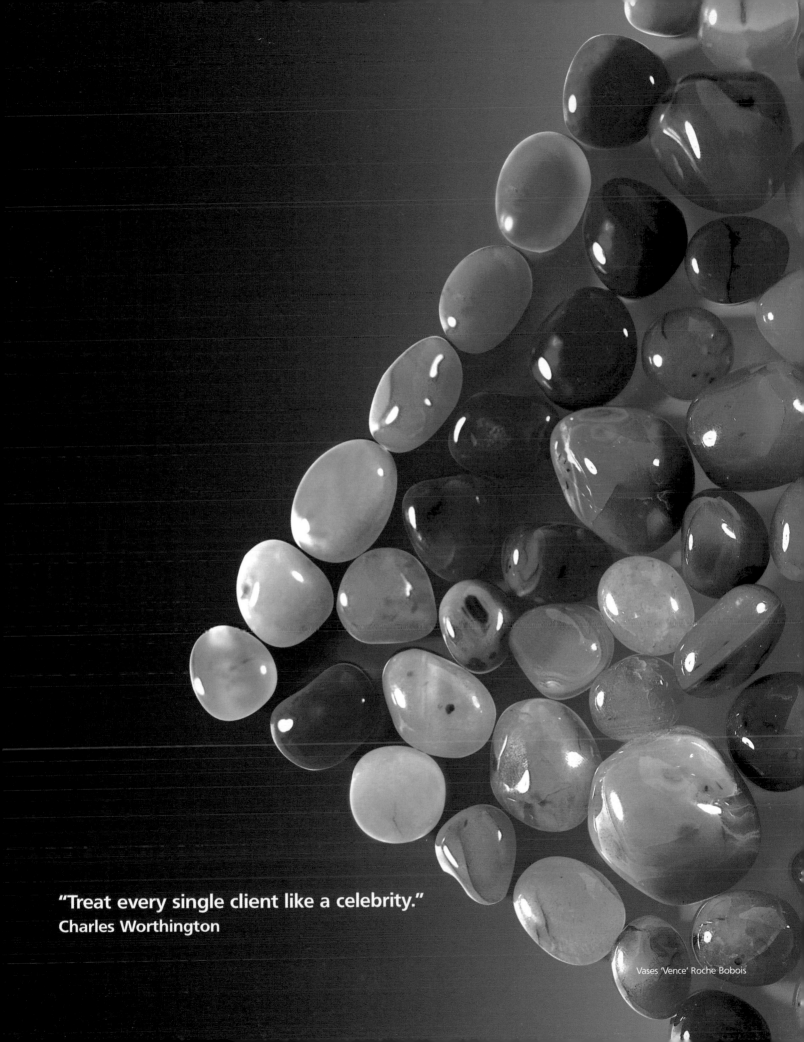

"Treat every single client like a celebrity."
Charles Worthington

Vases 'Vence' Roche Bobois

FEATHERED

This versatile technique combines effects from soft and delicate to bold and dramatic.

Step 1

Divide the hair into a side parting and take out a rectangular section across the crown.

Step 2

Using alternating products take back to back slices through this section.

Step 3

Make a full head colour application to the remaining hair.

Step 4

Develop in accordance with instructions.

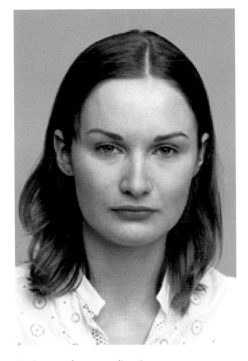

Before colour application

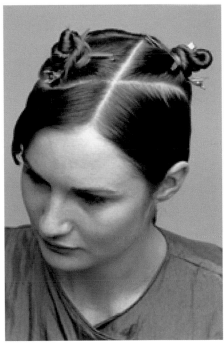

Step 1

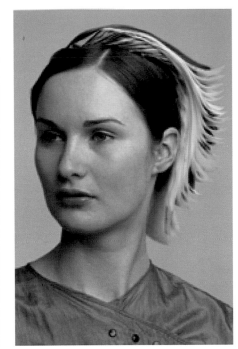

Step 2

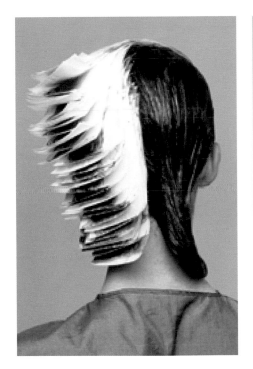

Step 3

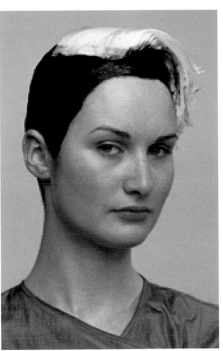

Step 4

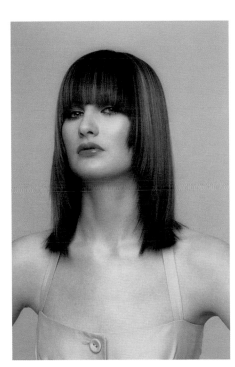

Final colour result

VERITY @ IMG Models

CRESCENT PIVOT

The crescent pivot technique is suitable for the mid-length to longer layered shapes.

Step 1

Make a crescent shaped section around the crown area.

Step 2

From the corner of the crescent section, make a triangular section down to the top of the ear and up to the front centre approx 2–3cm from the front hairline. Repeat on the other side making three zones in total.

Step 3

Work through each side section by taking diagonal slices with foils or Easi Meche up towards the centre parting. Use a large weave on the last two packets before the parting.

Step 4

Work diagonally across the final crescent shape section using a large weaving technique.

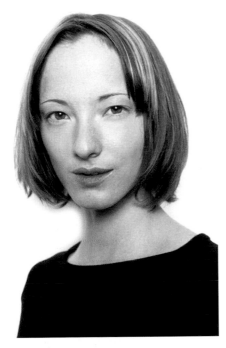

Before colour application

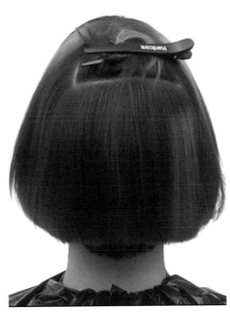

Step 1

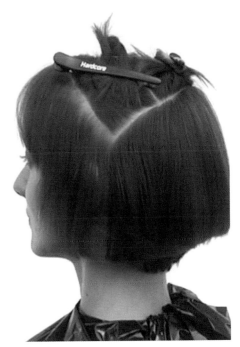

Step 2

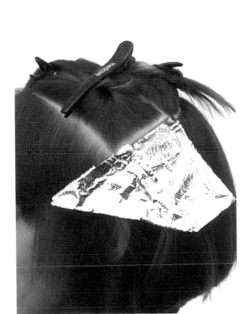

Step 3

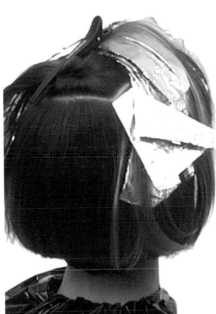

Step 4

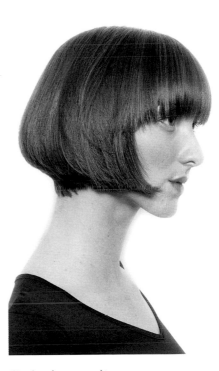

Final colour result

Toni & Guy International Technical Team

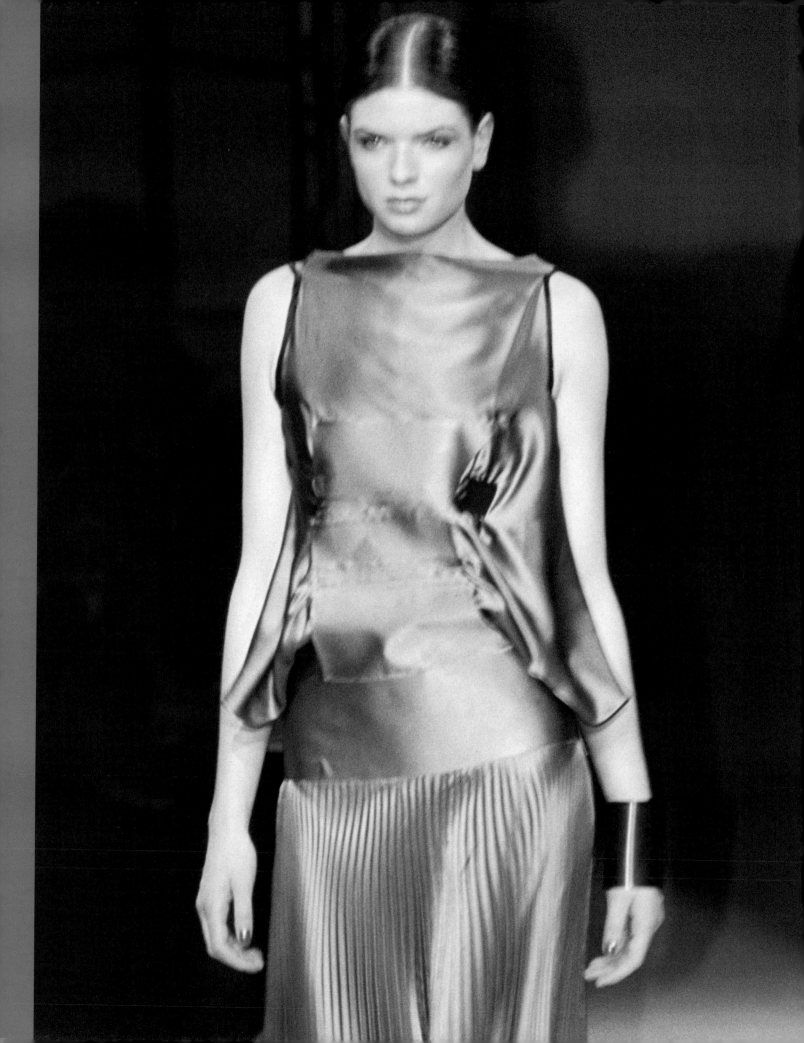

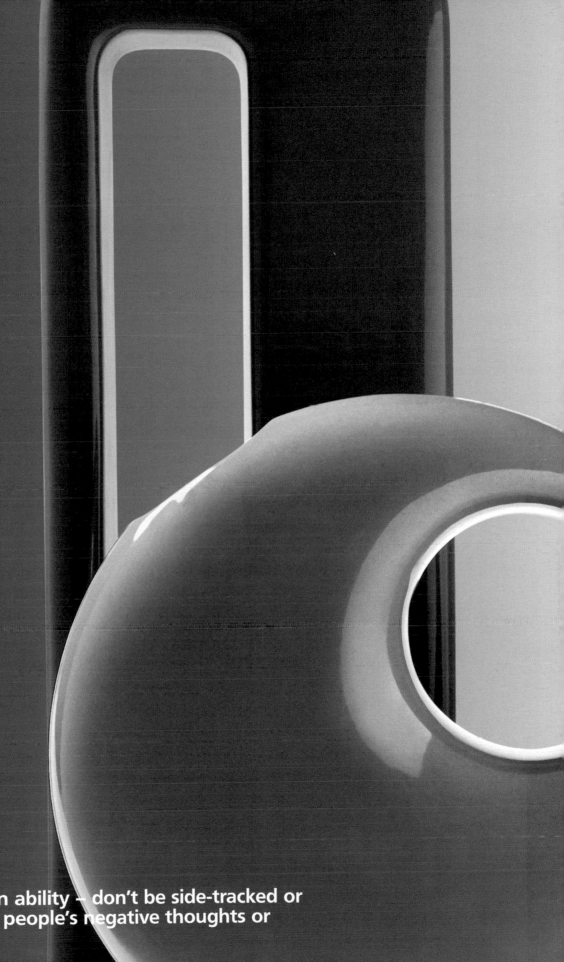

"Believe in your own ability – don't be side-tracked or influenced by other people's negative thoughts or comments."
Jo Hansford

Vases 'Vence' Roche Bobois

PLAITED

This technique creates a marbled effect and a diffused tone on thick, course and curly hair.

Step 1

Divide the hair into rectangles, make four sections across the top and two at each side.

Step 2

Separate the remaining hair at the back into four sections and loosely plait each section, backcombing ends to secure.

Step 3

Sub divide the top rectangles and plait the central part, plait side sections.

Step 4

On the remaining hair make slices using a lightening product. To the plaited hair sponge on a toning colour.

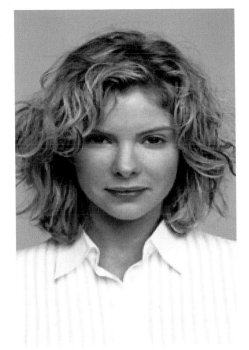

Before colour application

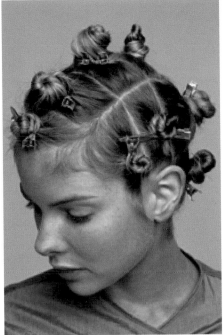

Step 1

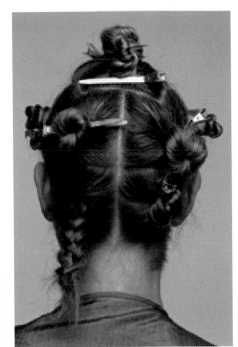

Step 2

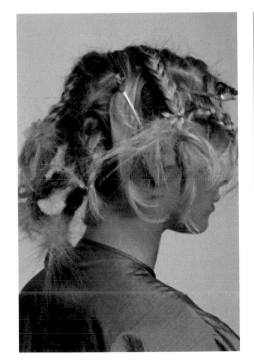

Step 3

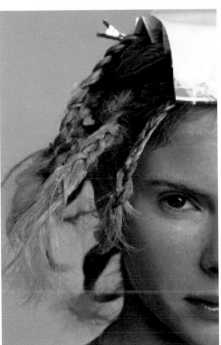

Step 4

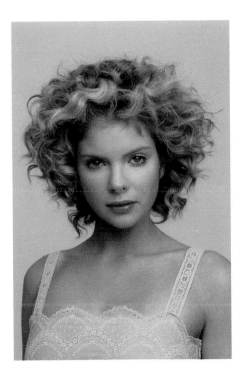

Final colour result

BRICK RADIAL

The brick radial technique is suitable for all lengths of layered hair.

Step 1

Take a halo section on the top of the head 2cm back from the front hairline.

Step 2

Starting at the front take a slice 1–2cm wide below the halo and seal in foil or Easi Meche, continue to work around the halo in this method.

Step 3

Take another halo section 2cm above the first. Using a brickwork pattern continue to take slice sections and work around the head.

Step 4

Continue to work upwards with the brickwork pattern until a small area is left on the top and then take slices through diagonally.

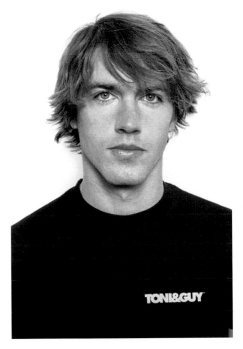

Before colour application

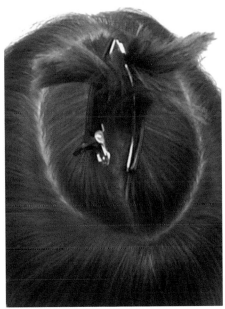

Step 1

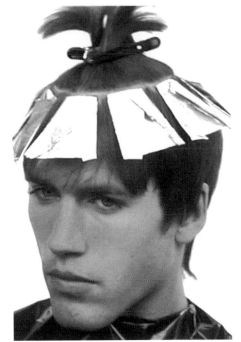

Step 2

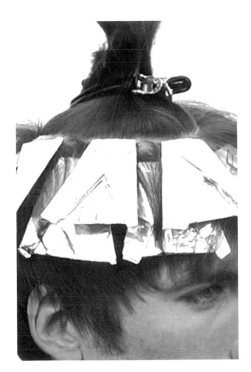

Step 3

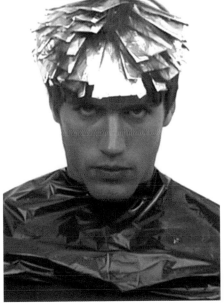

Step 4

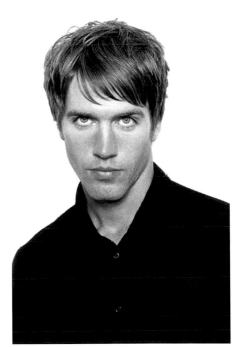

Final colour result

Toni & Guy International Technical Team

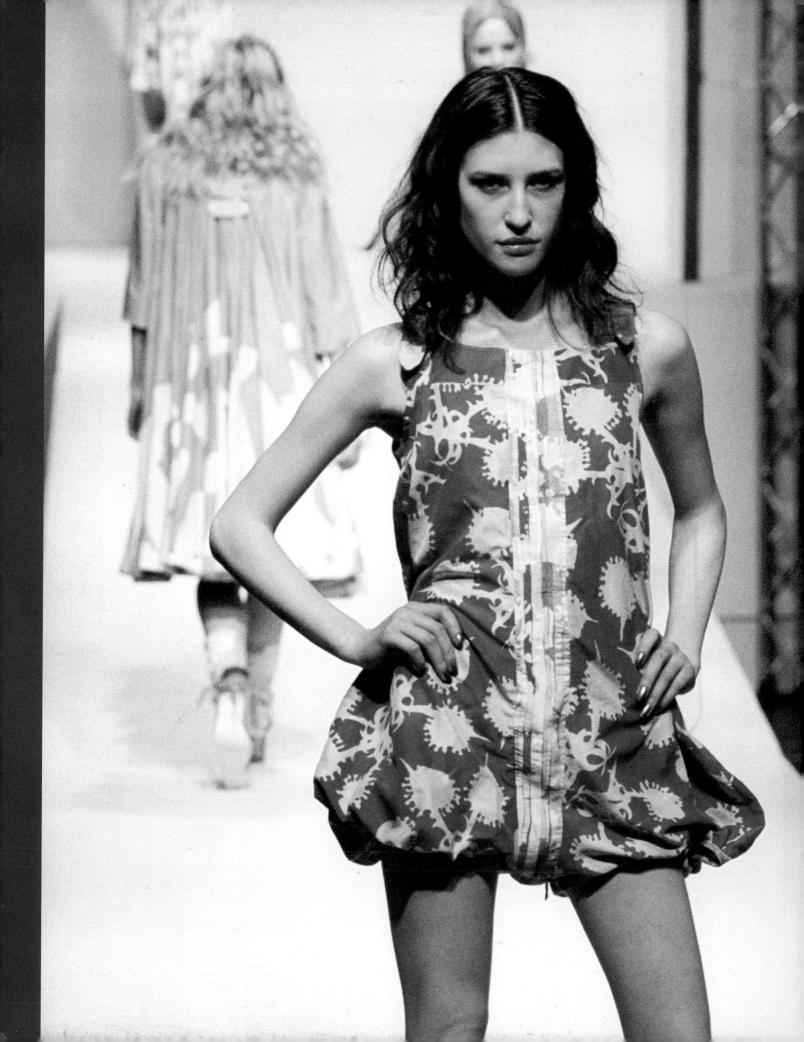

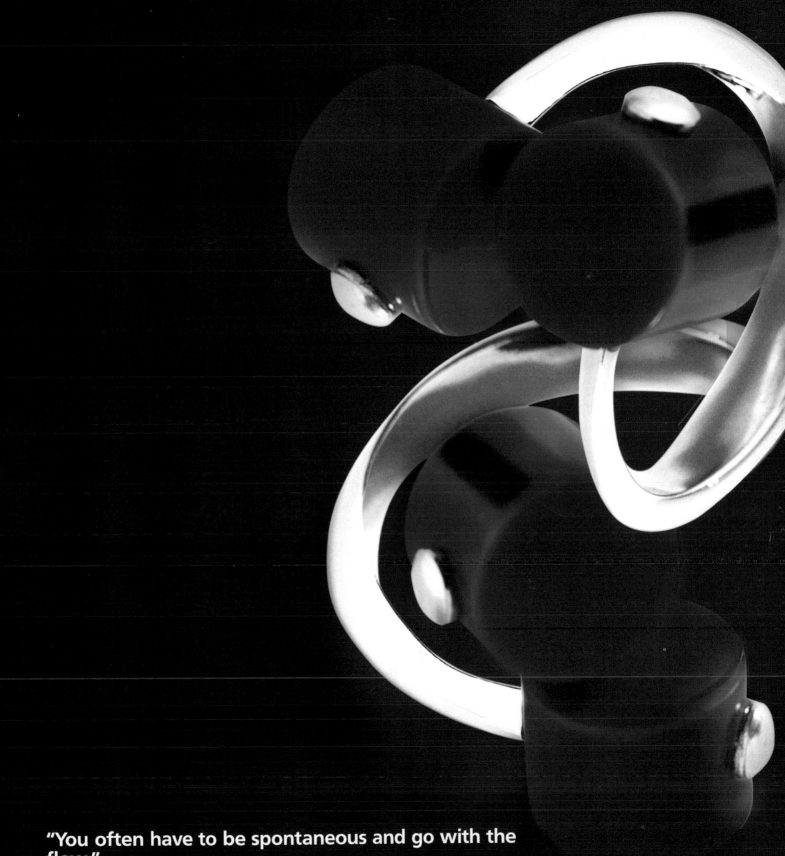

"You often have to be spontaneous and go with the flow."
Carly Alpin

Furla

ALTERNATIVE HALF HEAD

The alternative half head technique is suitable for medium to long layered shapes.

Step 1

Take a parting just below the crown to the top of the ear on both sides. Next take a triangular section from the top of the head to the high recession area, separate the triangle by taking a parting halfway along the diagonal to front. This now makes four sections in total.

Step 2

Taking diagonal sections, work through the side sections using a large weave and isolate in foils or Easi Meche.

Step 3

On the larger section at the front, take diagonal slice sections and work through.

Step 4

On the remaining section, use a large weaving technique to work through.

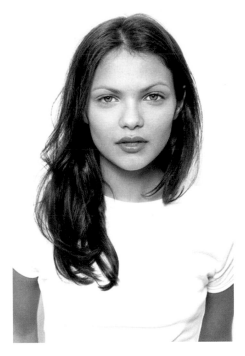

Before colour application

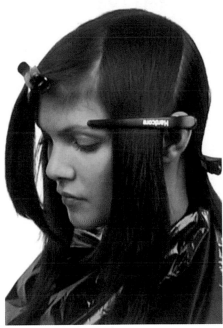

Step 1

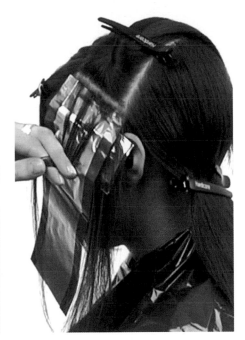

Step 2

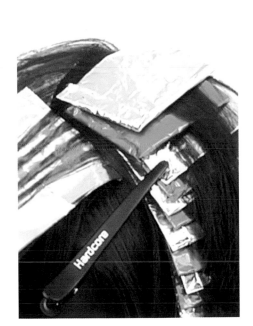

Step 3

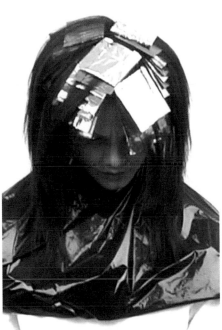

Step 4

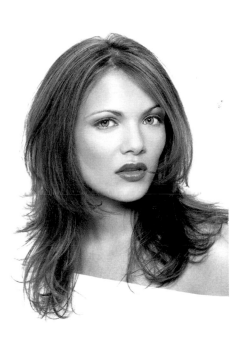

Final colour result

Toni & Guy International Technical Team

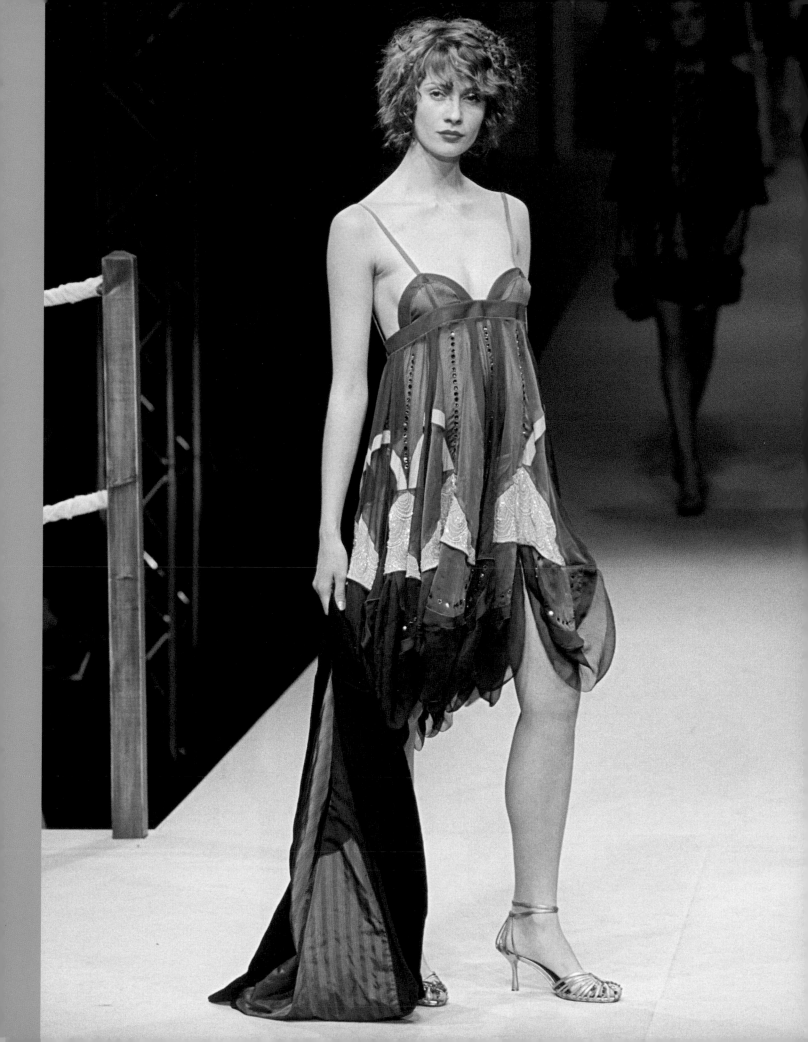

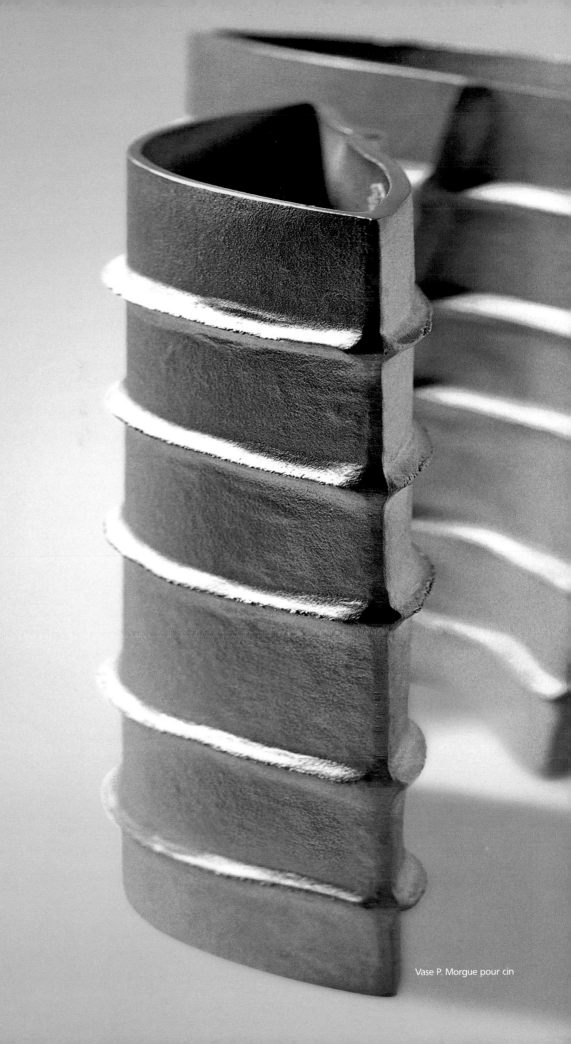

Vase P. Morgue pour cin

index